The
ENNEAGRAM
of
EATING

The ENNEAGRAM *of* EATING

How the 9 Personality Types
Influence Your Food, Diet, and
Exercise Choices

ANN GADD

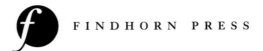
FINDHORN PRESS

Findhorn Press
One Park Street
Rochester, Vermont 05767
www.findhornpress.com

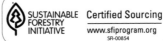

Text stock is SFI certified

Findhorn Press is a division of Inner Traditions International

Disclaimer
The information in this book is given in good faith and is neither intended to
diagnose any physical or mental condition nor to serve as a substitute for informed
medical advice or care. The author of this book does not dispense medical
advice nor prescribe the use of any food or technique as a form of treatment for
medical problems. Please contact your health professional for medical advice and
treatment. Neither author nor publisher can be held liable by any person for any
loss or damage whatsoever which may arise directly or indirectly from the use of
this book or any of the information therein.

A CIP record for this title is available from the Library of Congress

ISBN 978-1-62055-827-0 (print)
ISBN 978-1-62055-828-7 (ebook)

Printed and bound in the United States by Lake Book Manufacturing, Inc.
The text stock is SFI certified. The Sustainable Forestry Initiative® program promotes
sustainable forest management.

10 9 8 7 6 5 4 3 2 1

Edited by Nicky Leach
Text design, layout and illustrations by Damian Keenan
This book was typeset in Adobe Garamond Pro and Calluna Sans with
ITC Century Std used as a display typeface.

To send correspondence to the author of this book, mail a first-class letter to the
author c/o Inner Traditions • Bear & Company, One Park Street, Rochester, VT
05767, and we will forward the communication, or contact the author directly at
www.anngadd.co.za

Dedication

Thank-you seems such a small offering for all that I have
received, but here goes:

To those who have walked the precarious path between
weight gain and loss and whose comments weave their
way through this book. Heartfelt thanks.

To all the teachers who have inspired my learning,
in particular those early teachers who had the courage to
first share this wisdom with the world so more of us could
benefit from its insights, I am hugely grateful.

And to the Enneagram itself.

I never realized when I first idly picked up *The Wisdom
of the Enneagrams* (Riso/Hudson) all those years ago,
what a great and exciting journey awaited me and as a
result, how my understanding of self and others would
deepen so profoundly. As a regular workshop junkie,
I felt in the Enneagrams, I had at last found a path that
worked for me. I hope you'll find the same.

Contents

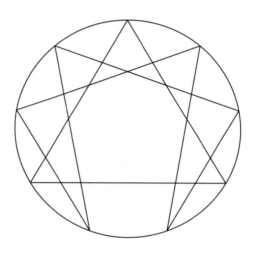

Prologue

I was born thin—so much so that my ribs protruded more than my breasts. In fact, if the measurement around my ribs was a 34C, then my breasts were a 34A. Sadly, I never appreciated my slim body and, as is the case with so many women, focused my feelings and low self-worth on my lack of meaningful breasts.

I maintained my 54-kilo weight until having my first child. From there it was a sticky bun slide downhill, from 55 to 100 kilos in 30 years. No cookies barred.

To reverse the steady accumulation of kilos, over the years I acquired a library of diet books, CDs, and seldom used gym equipment.

- The "eat only protein" diet.
- The "eat according to your blood type" diet.
- The "eat the way the French do" diet.
- The gluten-free diet.
- The "listen to tapes and that will kill your desire to eat" diet.
- The dietitian's "sensible eating plan" (you are *not* to use the word "diet").
- The "cut out all fats" diet.
- The "eat as much fat as you like" diet (but avoid carbohydrates and sugar).
- The "count the calories/kilojoules intake" diets.
- The cabbage soup diet.
- The coffee diet (my personal favorite).
- Protein shakes.
- Slimming drops.
- Pills to remove your appetite.
- Green tea.
- Herbal drinks (I was an agent).
- Yerba mate tea (and yes, it does taste foul).

- Weight loss clubs.
- Curves.
- Sure Slim.
- Personal trainers.
- Exercise routines.
- Swimming 50–100 lengths daily in a 50-meter pool.
- Walking 50 kilometers a week.
- Windsurfing (that really worked, but when motherhood and work demands curtailed activity the weight came pouring back).

I endlessly tried new trends and ideas in the fight against flab. The only reward for all that effort? An extra kilo or two annually.

My bookshelves creaked with advice from various authorities. I waded through volumes as each author expounded about their newfound dieting or "eating plan." Granted, many of them did show impressive images of their "before and after" figures, or those of their followers, while despite various attempts at losing weight, my body remained the same weight in my "before" photo as the "after" one. In fact, even though a slight weight loss may occasionally have occurred, within months it had crept back on.

The weight I had disliked 10 years ago now became my goal weight as I attempted yet another diet fad. I watched as friends, using one product or another, slimmed down dramatically, only to expand with even faster speed when they stopped taking the shake, slurping down endless bowls of cabbage soup, popping pills, or subscribing to an "eating plan."

I had read that most diets fail hopelessly in the long term and that in 83 percent[1] of cases, weight gain over and above the starting weight is the norm after a year. I had given up on myself, as I suspect many overweight people have.

As a result, I attempted the New Age thinking that I must learn to "love myself as I am." Not easy when you look in the mirror and see there is so much more of you to love than you feel good about loving. Success in all other aspects of my life was abundant, yet having spent half my life as a thin person, the weight gain in the second half of my life haunted me daily and ate voraciously at my self-esteem.

About the Enneagram

I was listening to the radio today and heard a woman complaining. She was on a strict diet of no sugar, high protein, and little or no carbohydrates while her office colleague ate stacks of french fries, daily footlong bratwurst hotdogs swimming in sugar-loaded tomato sauce and mustard, and sodas and a variety of sugary snacks in between. Despite this, her colleague remained skinny, while the caller's weight seemed to ignore her efforts entirely and stayed in its wobbly place.

I want to give you an insight into why that might be, so that you can view yourself and your desire to lose weight not just being about eating less but understanding that subconscious programming has told your body to desperately hold onto each kilogram, despite your conscious efforts. Key to that understanding is knowing your Enneagram personality type.

The Enneagram is a way of coming to a deeper understanding about ourselves and others. The insights provide a unique path for us to shed that which is not serving us and to realize the true nature of our being.

Gaining an understanding of your relationship to food as dictated by your Enneagram personality type will allow you to develop greater awareness about what underlies your eating habits and make better dietary choices to support your physical and emotional health.

Type "diet books" in your search engine, and Google alone brings up 159 million sites, while Amazon.com currently lists 53,000+ diet books available. That's a huge number of books, none of which can claim 100 percent success for most of their readers long term (or we'd all be skinny).

Dieting and its related products—shakes, pills, shelves of "low/no fat" foodstuffs, equipment, books, CDs, clothing in the form of "skinny jeans," and so on—have become seriously big business, making massive dollars, particularly for pharmaceutical companies and food brands. Yet despite this vast diet product infrastructure for the most part we remain overweight and globally are getting fatter while the producers of these goods gain financially.

It's a gain/gain situation … only one half of the gainers are not happy. It is estimated that in the USA alone 70.2 percent[1] of the population is overweight and roughly 30 percent of those are classified as obese. The impact this has on health is extreme, while manufacturers of all those diet pills double their profits selling additional healthcare remedies to people suffering from adult onset diabetes, high cholesterol, and other effects of being overweight. Moreover, the incidence of obesity is steadily increasing, with the most rapid rate of morbid obesity occurring in the 15–20-year-old age group.

Australia too has lumbered onto the broad bandwagon, where it is described as an epidemic. According to the *Medical Journal of Australia*, obesity had doubled in the country in the two decades prior to 2003.[2] Now two out of every three adults are overweight and over 25 percent are classified as obese.

Somehow, despite volumes of research and a plethora of new diet products, information, and foods being introduced into the marketplace, we simply aren't getting it (or getting too much of it!). We are, in a sense, killing ourselves with food, and we seem unable to stop eating. There may be valid reasons for weight gain, such as hormone imbalances, slow metabolism, and stress, but bottom line—we are clearly eating too many of the wrong types of foods. But why do certain programs/diets work for some people and not others?

Enter the Enneagram Types

I started studying the nine different Enneagram personality types roughly 14 years ago. Eight years later, completely fascinated by the subject, I am teaching them myself.

I had this aha! moment one day. I realized that the people writing the diet books or creating the eating plans are doing so based on their own personality type and their own personal level of stress. So if you aren't the same personality type or at the same developmental level as the author, chances are, you literally aren't on the same page.

As I delved deeper into the Enneagram personality types and discovered their many riches in terms of self-awareness, I realized that each personality type has a completely different approach to eating and, as a result, only certain methods will work for certain people.

I grabbed all the dusty volumes of diet books off my shelves and started to find a pattern. Different people/personalities put on weight for different reasons; therefore, losing weight will be greatly assisted by understanding these different reasons in depth, as well as looking at their emotional causes.

For instance, one author wrote that the "fight-or-flight" factor is the reason people gain weight. His thinking was that you either gain weight to appear larger to fend off the enemy or you lose it fast, so you can run away and escape at speed. This might fit "fear" type personalities but not necessarily those exhibiting "shame or guilt," so as a result, his book then would strike a chord with certain personalities, but not all.

It occurred to me that different people gain weight for different reasons, and until we get to the bottom of those reasons and work with them, the problem will continue. To coin a phrase from one of my teachers, Rosalyn Bruyere, it's like putting "whipped cream on garbage"—a success in the short term but not effective long term. This is why people may lose weight on a diet, but if the underlying emotional cause of the weight gain remains, they are destined to gain back the weight, just as taking a tranquilizer may reduce anxiety in a person at that moment but will not take away the reason they were anxious long term.

I attempted to investigate this mind/big body connection with various dietitians and people who work in weight management programs, but while many of them acknowledged that there was a link, they were, for the most part, not inclined to investigate further, as it was out of their knowledge realm.

The nine Enneagram personality types have been described by the Enneagram author and teacher Russ Hudson as "The Passage to Power."[3] As such, they are a path back to whole/holy ness and far more than the simple personality profiling system many people believe them to be. The nine primary Enneagram types diversify into others in many ways, but for the purposes of this book, we will stick with the nine primary types.

I started profiling the Enneagram personality types of the authors of each of the diet books in my library. In some cases it was a dead giveaway, while others were harder to pin down. It became clear, though, that for the most part each author was (perfectly understandably) writing for their Enneagram personality type. It follows then that by understanding the nine Enneagram personality types, we can become aware of our subconscious programming and be more specific about what is driving our food choices at different levels of health/stress. I reasoned that if certain weight loss books and CDs had worked, then it might be because they had connected with the Enneagram personality type of the author and reader.

Using my Enneagram knowledge, I profiled the approaches to eating of each of the nine Enneagram personality types, then, using these profiles as well as my previous work as an alternative healer and counselor, I was able to understand the emotional reasons why each type would put on weight, and more importantly, how to work with that information to help someone to reduce weight.

What will inspire and work for Enneagram Type One will have the opposite effect for Enneagram Type Seven, but if you can determine which Enneagram personality type you are, you can work with clearing out the garbage, avoid the whipped cream on top, and become healthier and happier. You will be working *with* yourself as opposed to *against* yourself.

Knowledge, as they say, is power. Knowing yourself on a deeper level, via the nine Enneagram personality types, will help you to understand your food choices, your approach to exercise, your potential addictions, as well as a range of habits relating to these and broader patterns of behavior. You will understand why you gain weight, what triggers your cravings and, using the information, be able to choose a weight loss plan suited to your personality.

No Gain Without Pain

This is not a diet book that's going to request that you ditch chocolate for the dubious delights of lentils. However, insight into yourself and why you are those few kilos overweight is not necessarily going to be pain free; when we examine ourselves—our emotional selves, that is—we must face not only the pleasant sides of ourselves but also those aspects we'd rather avoid. Nevertheless, seeing these aspects, and moreover, accepting them, makes you more conscious of who you are and, as a result, more able to gain insight into the inner, less conscious workings of your mind.

Doing introspective work takes courage because our natural reaction when we confront something about ourselves we don't like is to deny it. It's our ego's way of protecting itself. So be aware of strong emotions that may arise when you read the book, and even if you want to deny the feelings they evoke in you, do spend at least a short time reflecting on your life and whether this could be an aspect of yourself you don't want to see.

You may identify primarily with a certain type, yet be confused by seeing aspects of other types within you. It may feel like: *What? I'm sort of a Type Nine, but maybe also a Type Six, and Seven is also possible. How can that be? Maybe I'm mixed up?* This is because we all relate to all other types, some more than others.

For example, let's take Kate, a Type Six. You'll learn more about Type Six later, but for this exercise, the quick overview of a Six reveals it to be a fear-based personality that is part of what is known as the Thinking Triad. Sixes are loyal, responsible, compassionate, hard-working, ambivalent, anxious, can have issues with trust (themselves and others), engaging, generally have a good sense of humor, foresee possible problems, and in spite of their fear-based personality, can dig deep and become paradoxically very courageous, when required.

The fear fixation that is part of Kate's Enneagram personality type may lead her to try to maintain order through repetitive behaviors. This could be mistaken for Type One's desire for perfection through orderliness; however, Kate is seeking order to stave off her fear of chaos, while Type One is creating order because it's the "right thing to do."

As with many Sixes, Kate can become depressed, and this can be mistaken for the melancholy of Type Four.

Feeling unmotivated, she can become hugely procrastinating like a less healthy Type Nine.

To overcome this, Kate might then throw herself into studies and projects in a similar way to a Type Three (feeling shame when she fails to complete them—shame is part of a Three's experience).

When healthy, her compassion and empathy for others can feel to them as if they are with a loving Type Two.

When fear threatens to overcome her, she may try to throw caution to the wind, like an adventurous Type Seven, to prove to herself that she is not afraid moving to her Seven wing, (this could also be being a counter-phobic Type Six).

When this becomes too scary, she may retreat away from these feelings into her head and the safety of her own space and thoughts, much the same as a Type Five would do.

So you can see that Kate, although occasionally displaying traits of the other numbers (and no doubt, being able to relate to them) still maintains the fixation or motivation of a Type Six.

It is not my intention in this book to explain the entire Enneagram personality type system in depth. There are many wonderful books that do just that, some of which I have listed at the end of the book. However, if you know nothing about the Enneagram personality types, you may want to read this section to get a basic understanding of the system, which is the path from an ego-fixated self to essence. It is an amazing tool for self-awareness, a bit like having a book written especially for you in order to assist you in your personal growth.

When I teach the Enneagram system, a common reaction from my students is, "I don't want to be put in a box." That's the point, though: you are already in a box of your own personality's making. The constrictions we impose upon ourselves through our beliefs, fears, and fixations are not our true selves; they are just a poor and distorted reflection of our potential. The Enneagram is a way of breaking free from the box. To use a business cliché: it's a way of not only thinking out of the box but living outside of it.

One of the biggest traps in the Enneagram is to fall in love with your type and as a result, not feel the inclination to explore life outside its constricted view of the world. I so often hear people new to the Enneagram saying with great pride and glee, "I'm a Nine (or any other type)," as if that was an achievement within itself. The point is not to just find your box, but to liberate yourself from it and in so doing move beyond your type and its fixations. Doing so takes much inner work, because it's not the brilliant integrated aspects of our type that grow us as much as becoming conscious of the less healthy aspects.

To transcend to the next level of our being means to sit with, for example, the side of ourselves that feels a failure on one hand, with the need to appear hugely successful on the other. Only when we can be okay with failure and success, can we transcend the need to be either. Then we can shift from being invested in keeping the failure hidden whilst waving flags to get acknowledgement for our successes.

It's not uncommon to mistype or be mistyped. Personally, the type I originally thought I was turned out not to be my actual type after all. In fact, I moved through several types before I 'found' myself. I don't regret it though, because living through the eyes of those other types gave me huge insight into these types and led me to experience more of the whole Enneagram. If unsure, go with whatever type draws you (or maybe even with the one that least attracts if nothing strikes a cord).

The Basics

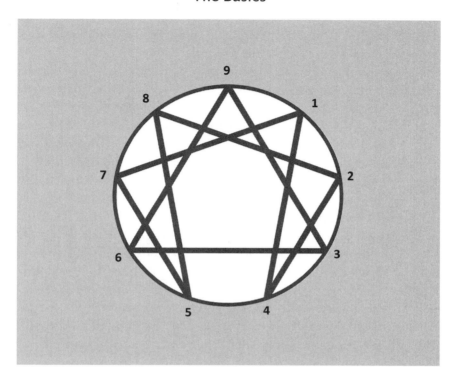

The Enneagram consists of nine basic personality types, which can then be divided further into various three-way divisions, resulting in many other sub-types. The nine equidistant points which you see on the circle diagram represent the nine basic types. Each of us is born as one type, which remains constant throughout our lives.

The types give us insight into how we navigate the world. Our type is not formed by our youth, but rather, one could say, our childhood is formed by our type. This means that children of certain types will experience similar types of experiences (not necessarily in the way they manifest but issues such as feeling overlooked or growing up in a conflict-ridden household).

The types are relevant irrespective of sex, race, or any other possible dividing factor, so a Type Six as a male tribal member in Africa will have a similar emotional/mental makeup to a Type Six woman living in the USA. (That's one of the things I love about the Enneagrams: it unites us across continents and all divides.)

There is no hierarchy in the Enneagrams. A Type One is no better or worse than an Eight or any other types, for instance. We all have our strengths and weaknesses, although the form they take is different. Each type has lessons to learn and issues to work through.

The symbol itself consists of a circle, a triangle, and an irregular hexagram. How the various points connect is a very important aspect of the Enneagram but beyond the scope of this book. Suffice it to say that if you see the point Four, for instance, you will see that it connects through the inside lines to both the Two and One points. This means that if you're a Type Four, you may display traits of both the numbers your number connects with, that is, Type Two and Type One, or alternatively, as a Type Three, you'll connect to aspects of a Type Nine and Type Six.

The lines between the points are sometimes known as the "Direction of Integration (Growth) and Disintegration (Stress)", see Russ Hudson/ Don Riso - Enneagram Institute. The iEQ9 (Integrated 9 Enneagram Solutions) calls them the "Journey of Stretch or Release." Other schools, authors and teachers have alternative names, but the meaning is essentially the same; namely that the numbers that are connected to the type, have an influence on the type or can potentially influence that type. Thus, your type is not simply a static point but is a point on a moving energetic flow around the symbol.

To use the iEQ9 terminology, the "release" line for Type Three would be to a Type Six and the "stretch" line would be towards Type Nine. For a Type Four, release would be towards a Type One and stretch towards Type Two. Moving towards a stretch number usually provokes change but can prove to be harder, whereas moving towards a release point usually releases tension and stress. This movement is just one reason that you can find aspects of yourself in different types.

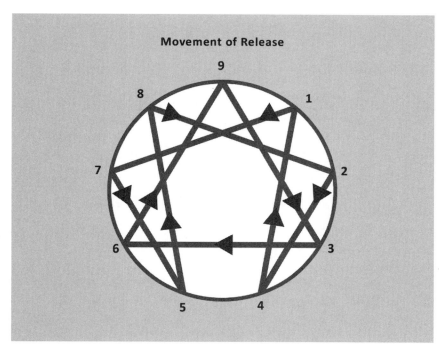

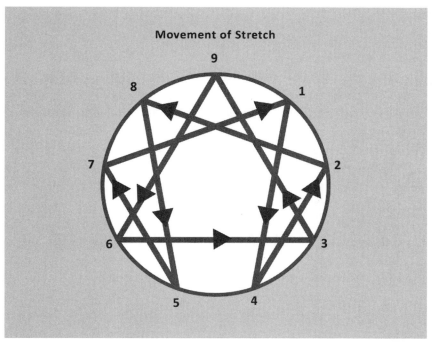

The Three Centers

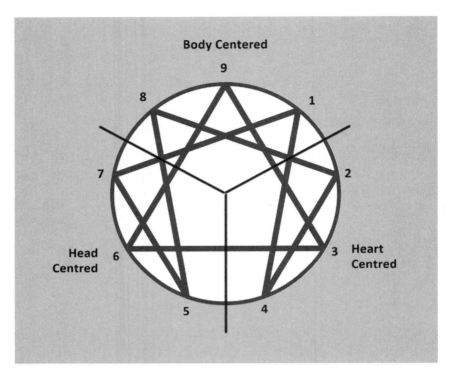

The Enneagram can be divided into several groups of three. The grouping of *Instinctual/Body*, *Feeling/Heart*, and *Thinking/Head* types is of prime importance. (Note: The *Instinctual/Body* center must not be confused with *Instinctual Types*, which are discussed farther on in this section.) It does not mean that a Feeling Type does not have anger or that a Thinking Type has no feelings; it means that they have issues in these fields. Whether they show up as strengths or weaknesses will depend on the emotional / mental health of each individual.

This further translates into Instinctual Types having issues with or particular lessons to learn from anger, Feeling Types with shame, and Thinking Types with fear. These "fixations" form the core wounding of each triad and may be viewed as the stumbling block of each type when they are personality or ego focused.

Much of the Enneagram is based on the Law of Three[4]: an active expression, a passive expression, and a neutral/combining/balancing between the two expressions and the Law of Seven.[5] This is indeed a fascinating dimension and expression of the Enneagrams, and I recommend further reading.

WINGS – The Numbers on Either Side of Each Personality Type

For the purposes of this book, we occasionally need to distinguish between an Enneagram personality type's "wings" as they relate to diet or exercise.

So what is a wing? Basically, your wings are the numbers on either side of your Enneagram personality type (so if you're a Type Six you could have a Five or Seven wing, or if you are a Nine you may have a One or Eight wing). These wings influence your personality type. Think of it like shifting hues. Add red to yellow, and the red will give a warmer, more orange hue. Add green to yellow, and the green will give a cooler, more lime shade. However, the color remains essentially yellow. For example, a Type Nine with an Eight wing will be more inclined to be heavy like a typical Eight, rather than leaner if they have a One wing.

While some people may have both wings, it's more common for one of them to dominate. As a result, a Type Four with a Five wing will appear different to a Four with a Three wing. Wings and their relative strengths can alter in our lifetimes. Once you have determined your type, it's easier to ascertain what (if any) wing is dominant.

INSTINCTUAL VARIANTS – The Three Instinctual Preferences Found in Each Type

Within each Enneagram personality type are three instinctual preferences referred to as Self-Preservation, Social, or Sexual.[6] The order of importance of these three instincts in each type plays an important role in creating differences within the types and the one of least importance provides an area of potential growth. These instinctual variants relate back to our basic instincts, which may have had the emphasis distorted according to our childhood environment.[7]

These are our basic animal instinctual drives. They are similar to the first three layers of Maslow's Hierarchy of Needs. 1) Physiological needs—warmth, shelter, rest, food (Self-Preservation); 2) Safety and Security needs (Social—being part of a tribe or pack ensures the safety of the individual); and 3) Love and Friendships needs (Sexual—the need to create one-on-one relationships and enjoy intimate contact).

In the Enneagram, the Self-Preservation Instinct focuses on survival needs and our general well-being (physiological and safety). The Social

Instinct is how we navigate the connections we create with others and our communities. The Sexual Instinct focuses on the drive to create one-on-one chemistry and intimacy with another.

The instinct that tops our list will be where we devote too much energy, and the least important will be where we focus little effort. A personality develops based on our Enneagram type's fixation and basic fears.

Having similar instinctual types in our relationships can go a long way to helping us understand each other. It stands to reason that if one person is focused on work and earning (Self-Preservation) while the other seeks intimate connection (Sexual Instinct), not understanding the other's Instinctual needs could create frustration and misunderstanding.

Self-Preservation Instinct: Your focus is drawn more toward navigating the basic physical needs in life, such as earning an income, food, comfort, having a safe home, and self-preservation, in general (or in primal terms, hunting, gathering, and fighting off enemies).

Social Instinct: Your focus is on navigating social groups or tribes to preserve your safety and ensure tribal survival. For many animals, being ousted from the group results in a much greater mortality rate. It does not mean that you are necessarily wildly social; rather, you are concerned with and value group interaction. You will enjoy working for the good of the community and may belong to committees and groups where social responsibility is the key motivation. It's safety in numbers!

Sexual Instinct: You are not necessarily wildly sexually active, but your focus is on forming intimate bonds with others (which also secures the future of the tribe). It can translate as enjoying the stimulation or buzz of connecting with someone new, even if there is no sexual attraction—it's the excitement of the energy between you and another person that you enjoy. It stands to reason then that Sexual types are more intense, electric, and charged-up than the other types.

LEVELS OF HEALTH – Your Emotional/Mental Health

As each personality type becomes more stressed, they will become less emotionally healthy. There is also a chance that their physical health will be affected, as stress is the main precursor to all illness. Also, the less healthy you are, it figures that the poorer your choices will be in all aspects of life, because your programming says you don't deserve better. The terminology for the Riso/Hudson range of behaviors is Healthy, Average, and Unhealthy.[8]

In their book, *Personality Types*, Russ Hudson and Don Richard Riso identified nine Levels of Development (LoD) (three under each heading). For the purposes of this book, it's sufficient to say that there are three main levels. These levels of health can change by the minute, day, or years, as we integrate and disintegrate.

Seeing Yourself in More than One of the Types

The Enneagram is a very complex system, and it's not my intention to cover all those aspects in this book. This book is essentially about our approach to eating and understanding our relationship to food, food choices, entertaining, diet, and exercise.

While we are fundamentally one type, we can show aspects of certain other types within the Enneagram framework. As a result, you may see aspects of your approach to eating in more than one type.

Do You Change Types During Your Lifetime?

The answer is no. While it's normal to move up and down the healthy or unhealthy states as life unfolds, your type does not alter.

Personality Type Titles

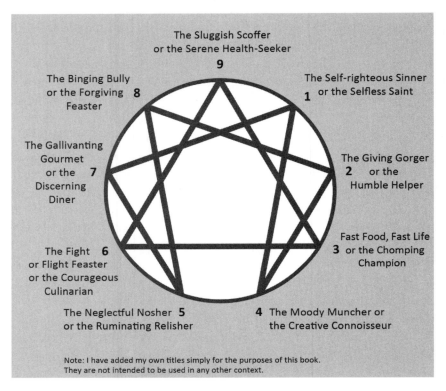

The Sluggish Scoffer
or the Serene Health-Seeker
9

The Binging Bully
or the Forgiving 8
Feaster

The Self-righteous Sinner
1 or the Selfless Saint

The Gallivanting
Gourmet
or the 7
Discerning
Diner

The Giving Gorger
2 or the
Humble Helper

Fast Food, Fast Life
3 or the Chomping
Champion

The Fight 6
or Flight Feaster
or the Courageous
Culinarian

The Neglectful Nosher 5
or the Ruminating Relisher

4 The Moody Muncher or
the Creative Connoisseur

Note: I have added my own titles simply for the purposes of this book.
They are not intended to be used in any other context.

I have used my own Enneagram titles for chapter headings. This is not because I want to detract in any way from the commonly used titles given by other authors, but because I wanted names specifically relating to the purpose of this book, for example, Diet, Eating, and Exercise. I feel that it's easier for the reader to identify with their eating patterns than the more generalized names.

It's also relevant to note that the names reflect our levels of health. So if we take the Type One chapter, which is entitled the Self-righteous Sinner or the Selfless Saint, then the view of ourselves as Sinner reflects the view of an average to unhealthy Type One, whereas Saint is more reflective of a healthy Type One.

We move through these levels of development or behavior throughout our lives, and even from day to day, so you could be most saintly in the morning when it comes to eating correctly, only to view yourself as a sinner under stress as you glug back wine and dive into the tapas.

Type One
The Self-Righteous Sinner or the Selfless Saint

The Issue

Type Ones strive for self-regulation, optimal body function, and a morally correct diet, but when the pressure of perfection builds too intensely, it results in an inner rebellion and does just the opposite. The pattern then becomes strict (holy) restraint in the pursuit of perfectionism, followed by secret binging, followed by intense remorse and an ever more intense need for self-discipline.

Overview of Type One

If you are a Type One, chances are you are not overweight (see exception under "How They View Their Bodies" on page 33). But you may *believe* you are, even when those close to you tell you otherwise, because Ones want to be beyond reproach. If perfectionism is relevant in your life, you would be harshly critical of any curve in the wrong place or lax eating habit on your part (or on the part of another). Whereas some of the other personality types may have a "live for the moment" attitude and worry about the consequences of overindulgence later (or never), the One truly wants to do what they believe is the right thing, and this includes their eating patterns, alcohol consumption, and exercise routine.

The need to be perfect translates into having high personal standards, with a strong moral overtone and conviction. While other personality types may be less than happy with their physical shape, for the One, the need to be perfect can completely dominate their lives, wreaking havoc with their health and emotions, as they seldom allow themselves to drop their guard and relax into simply being. They are trustworthy, rational, responsible, idealistic at times, fair, and have a great desire to improve not only themselves (and sometimes others) but also the world in general.

If a One has indulged and put on a few extra kilos on that long-awaited boat cruise, on their return, they will immediately implement a strictly disciplined regime to get back to their original weight. Ones are generally hard on themselves and will hold themselves to task if they feel they are not living up to their personally imposed ideals (which are typically very high). They do not approve of excess in any form, so unless it's a secret binge (which they can do to relieve the build-up of tension), as they move into the unhealthier levels of their being, Ones feel more comfortable remaining in control, when it comes to eating and drinking. They may also harshly judge others they see behaving inappropriately and overindulging.

Ones want to be good and do the right thing. They want to be role models in society. It's what gave them brownie points as children, so as adults they crave the same. The problem is that the issue of what is good and right varies from person to person, dietitian to doctor, and culture to culture. It's impossible to live up to all these expectations, so the One becomes like a hamster on a wheel—running in circles, putting vast amounts of energy into trying to get approval for doing the right thing, yet constantly feeling they've missed the mark. Ones may have a hidden desire to be someone great—the president, for example—occupying a role that they believe allows them to make meaningful changes in the world.

Ones are seldom open to change, believing that "If it ain't broke, don't fix it." Mind will rule over the heart in most cases. They may start many projects but not finish them, as to finish something means it would have to be finished perfectly. So afraid that it won't be perfect, they may feel more comfortable leaving the project unfinished. Ones are frugal rather than frivolous.

Occasionally, the need to repress their more instinctual nature can build up, leaking out into unexpected and out-of-control behavior, which may come as a surprise to both them and others. Less healthy Ones can be inflexible and judgmental, convinced that their "right way or truth" is THE right way or truth. Anger emerges in sudden vitriolic outbursts where they will not accept any form of criticism. They can become intolerant of others' views and lifestyles and have a narrow-minded worldview.

If they understand that they have disintegrated, Ones can work consciously to become the wise, kind, moderate, and accepting soul that is their potential.

Career Choices

Ones are good at organizing and detail work, so you'd find them typically as accountants, bookkeepers, office administration managers, head of the school parent-teachers association, treasurers, teachers, organizing charity events, or should they draw on that aspect of themselves that so clearly defines right from wrong, as church ministers, evangelists, Greenpeace workers, or in the legal world. They are conscientious and hard workers.

Eating Triggers

Warning signs that a Type One may be moving to less healthy behaviors would be having eating disorders, obsessive-compulsive disorders, increasing rigidity or inflexibility in their eating habits, as in "I know we're camping miles from anywhere, but I can only eat organic, freshly picked beets, even if you insist on eating canned goods." Here in the quote, you'll also see intolerance toward others' choices, with moral superiority added to the mix. Punishing behaviors may arise, such as subjecting themselves to endless cleanses and purges or forcing themselves to drink nasty tasting herbal concoctions, and so on.

When Type Ones feel they have been "bad" in some way, their all-or-nothing approach will have them swinging into a binging bonanza, all the while telling themselves they are not worthy of looking good. It's also a result of the tension within that builds because of the self-imposed pressure to be doing the right thing. Anger is expelled then in an act or acts of rebellion. If they feel they failed at doing it right, they may sabotage themselves by doing it very wrong.

How Ones Approach Eating

A regimented diet and discipline are the key words to describe a One's approach to eating. Ones have a very clear idea of what is right and wrong. Fat = wrong, skinny = right, unless they are an Eskimo or born in the 16th century and applying for the job as the artist Rubens' latest model!

Most of the time, a One will live according to a strict code of conduct and moral code, with a critical voice playing in their heads along the lines of, *It's wrong to be greedy. One helping is sufficient. Self-restraint is noble. Waste not, want not.* They may have been tempted in a moment of weakness to eat the entire pint of cookie dough ice-cream, but now the critic inside their head is going to make them pay for being so wicked. A purging of some sort may be the option (think of the ancient practice of self-flagellation so popular several centuries ago). A regimented diet, a fast, or the foregoing of what gives you pleasure in the food world will be the way a One could punish themselves when they do teeter over the edge into eating pleasure. Pills, fasts, fads, enemas, and a weird and bland choice of foods may all form part of this approach.

For the average One, life is a constant feeling of never quite living up to their own expectations of themselves and judging others for what they see as failing to do the same. As they become emotionally healthier, Ones will start to lighten up and become less harsh critics about all aspects of themselves.

Ones Eating Out

It's likely that the One type will be the first to arrive and if not early, then certainly punctually, because arriving on time is simply the right thing to do; this includes being irritated with others who arrive late. "Five minutes early is on time. Being on time is late," a Type One posted on Facebook. It gives hostesses like me the horrors. We are usually flinging on some clean clothes while adding the last ingredients to the dessert and trying to clean up some cat vomit when the doorbell rings early.

At the buffet table, most Ones will look at all the options and run their choice not through what they want to eat but rather what they "should" eat. They can view food choice as a path to whole(holy)ness and may opt to become vegan or vegetarian, motivated by the desire to be both morally and healthily "correct."

They may want to have the flaky-crust chicken pie in the creamy mushroom sauce, but their inner critic (often sounding like a parental voice) is telling them that it's loaded with fat, white flour, and battery-reared chicken and they would be much better off eating the chickpea and sprout salad.

Should someone else order what they perceive as being a healthier option, the One may find this annoying—they want to be seen as having the healthiest choice at the table. I've noticed Ones changing their order when they perceive that they haven't ordered the most holy(some) item on the menu. Today, for example, a One friend of mine WhatsApped an image of the pizza she was eating, then hastily added in a subsequent text that it was, in fact, gluten-free and had a cauliflower base with no cheese, just in case we thought she was being "bad."

Ones are also unlikely to pile food onto their plates. Restraint is usually the order of the day, and they may feel within their rights to comment adversely if they see someone with more than they believe is appropriate. Manners are important, both theirs and others.

Ones can be extremely fussy about what they eat and how it's prepared. "Are the vegetables organic and produced locally? Are you positive? Please ensure they are not overcooked. No salt please. I know the menu says 'pan fried,' but I'd like mine grilled. Are you sure this is grilled?" They may insist that the hot milk is not hot enough for their coffee, or that the fish isn't absolutely fresh.

I ate at a restaurant with a One once. Admittedly the food was badly prepared, but my dining companion sampled three dishes before finally (and grudgingly) settling on eating just some of the third dish. It's not that it's right to let restaurants get away with poor food or service; it's just that Ones can become overly picky, demanding, and opinionated in how the chef should have prepared their food.

Ones are not afraid to call to task those who they feel have wronged them. So if the waiter is not up to scratch or the food is badly prepared, it will most likely be the hard taskmaster One or the "don't mess with me" Eight telling them so. Of all the Enneagram types, they are the most likely to send back food in a restaurant.

When not eating in their own homes, where they can control the cleanliness, Ones may feel strongly about standards of cleanliness and the appropriate food preparation in the home they are visiting. This may even affect their decision as to where they will or won't eat ("I just can't eat at Sue's when I see the mess and clutter. I wonder just how long it's been since she actually gave the place a good cleaning. I worry about germs, so I'll eat only what came straight out of a packet").

Ones can be quite careful about parting with cash. While their need for scrupulous fairness will lead them to leave a tip, it will be perhaps not overly generous.

Ones Entertaining at Home

The table has been laid since 3 o'clock in the afternoon, even though the guests are only due at 7 p.m. The One has spent ages trying to decide whether to go for the classic "blue" look—blue placemats, cutlery with blue handles, blue napkins, the white crockery with a blue pattern, irises, and blue candles—or to go for the more sensual "red" look (the same, only with roses and red crockery). Ones are most likely, though, to have set ways of doing things when it comes to presentation. Everything is ordered and often storage places labelled. The decor will be neat, practical, and conservative.

Soon, recrimination creeps in. For example, "I should have written down what I prepared the last time the Barrows and Smiths came for dinner, then this time I could have made sure I made something else. Drat. A major slipup. I should really have invited the Watsons, but that would exceed the amount of my matching cutlery, so I'll have to invite them next time." "Are the table napkins too flash?" "Are the children's toys put away?" (And woe betide a child who doesn't lay the table correctly!)

The truth is, Ones often don't really enjoy cooking as much as they enjoy creating the perfect ambiance for their guests to experience. It's a tense experience following every detail of the recipe, and Type Ones will measure and weigh ingredients accurately. Chances are they may even do a trial run before the dinner, just to make sure they have things correctly done on the night. There will be enough food, but not the lavish helpings you might find at the home of some of the other types.

But even if cooking doesn't appeal to them, many Ones are good bakers and cake decorators. The precision required for both skills perfectly suits their nature. You seldom find a good baker who just tosses everything together and hopes for the best—weighing or measuring ingredients carefully is the answer to a successful outcome. (This may explain why I'm not the greatest baker!)

While the One fusses and creates ordered perfection, there is always this critical, judgmental voice telling her (or him) that she/he has failed to live up the to voice's expected standards. Afterwards, in her/his head, our One will go through the evening recriminating herself /himself for what she felt she should have done better, no matter how much people enthuse about the meal. She knows the filet was far from perfect and the wafers not quite crispy enough, while the beans were overdone. When will it ever be perfect? Ones hone in on the imperfections and ignore what did work.

With all this pressure, it's understandable that a One may simply decide it's all too much effort and entertain very little.

Should there be leftovers, Ones may be inclined to refrigerate them and use them at some later stage. They don't like throwing food away, seeing this as wasteful when so many hunger in the world. So they may hold onto food and may in some cases even eat beyond the sell by date of the food.

My dad was a One. He would insist on eating the old stale bread, when the dog would happily have eaten it, before he would use the new loaf.

This habit was undoubtedly made worse because of living through World War II and its food rationing, but years later, he never got over it. His favorite meal was a fry-up of all the leftover vegetables—the traditional British bubble and squeak.

Ones can become obsessed with cleanliness, which can manifest in food preparation and excessive washing up of utensils and cleaning countertops. I remember once having a very nice One to supper who told me that if she ever went to a house where a cat jumped onto a table, she would not eat at that house. As she was telling me this (and eating her roast lamb with relish), I watched in horror as my cat jumped on the kitchen counter behind her, in his ever-persistent search for butter. Some things are best left unsaid!

Food Choices

As a One, chances are you'll have gathered a vast amount of information on the "right" and "wrong" foods. Trouble is, new claims are being made almost daily about the benefits of various foods, as marketers push to get their products sold.

Ones will opt for the "right" choices rather than what may appeal to them. "I want a burger on a bun with pepper sauce, but will suppress this urge and opt for the lentil burger on a zucchini base, which I see as being a healthy option. I almost feel noble in this decision to opt for the good." It becomes then not about the enjoyment of the food but the enjoyment of the feeling of righteousness at choosing "good" food over "bad." Ones often enjoy healthy food, even if it's bland, because their enjoyment is mental rather than sensual.

Bland choices can also be a form of punishment for Type One, as well as proof that they can rise above their base instinctual desires. It's not only the actual food choice that is important to a One; it's also the moral choice. Free-range, grass-fed meat; organic produce; locally sourced food; and sustainable farming practices will all strongly influence a One.

Being a vegetarian or vegan offers a Type One the chance to be perfect in both body and mind, in terms of having no guilt about animals/the planet/deforestation or any of the issues related to eating meat. Inevitably, though, inner conflicts emerge as Ones want to eat soybeans rather than meat but if they eat non-organic soybeans (and corn) raised in the US these are almost all genetically modified, so they become obsessed with their food having to be labeled "organic" or "non-GMO." (*What is the right thing to do?*)

They are suspicious of their own bodily desires, so while they may want a certain food, they may not trust the pleasure a certain food could potentially offer.

When shopping, they will often have a list of items needed, so as not to be tempted to indulge in less healthy options. Scheduled meal plans for the week are common. They are thrifty and may not buy a certain item if it's seen as being overpriced, even if it was part of a planned meal. They tend to stick to the same brands and items.

Standing at the checkout till, Type Ones may feel that the person behind them in line is judging their choice of products, or they themselves may judge the contents of their fellow shoppers' carts *(Sweets and chocolates as well as frozen pies. When will people learn what's good for them?).*

This rigorous definition of "right" from "wrong" is also applied to the foods that Ones choose to eat. Depending on what diet, religious system, or food guru they are following, Ones can easily fall into the trap of labelling certain foods and drinks as "bad." I've known Ones to become increasingly bizarre in what they eat as they become less healthy. They will take pleasure in avoiding other more pleasurable foodstuffs and gain inner brownie points for doing so.

What You May Not See

Inside every Type One, there is a fun-loving, hedonistic Type Seven (Gallivanting Gourmet/Discerning Diner) wanting to break free. The less healthy Ones are emotionally and the more they judge themselves harshly, the greater the likelihood that this Seven side of themselves will emerge. This is why Ones can, particularly on holiday, break out and occasionally do something outrageous. Abusing alcohol on the quiet or having a one-night fling may be a way a less healthy One would relieve their inner tension.

I recall a One friend who was the epitome of righteousness in his working and home life. His wife was not like him at all, yet he would stoically and soberly observe her wild behavior without comment. Then one night, away from home, he suddenly started to strip and performed a wild gyrating dance as clothes flew in every direction. Anyone else aged 25 who acted like this would just have had a few too many beers, but coming from him, it was an astonishing performance. It was completely out of character—or as we now know, the pressure of always being good had reached its explosion point.

This hidden side of a One doesn't want to say no to the second glass of wine or refuse the double chocolate delight; in fact, this aspect of the One wants to taste the wine, vodka, and every cocktail on offer and round it off with a double cheeseburger and fries, plus whatever their repressed shadow side desires. Many Ones, though, may never access or acknowledge this hidden aspect of themselves.

Remember the pious mayor, Le Compte Paul de Reynaud, in the film and book *Chocolat* by Joanne Harris? He is convinced that the chocolate Easter delicacies that chocolatier Vianne has made for the village will make people stray from their faith in God, so he sneaks into her patisserie, with the idea that he will ruin all of her Easter goodies. After tasting a morsel of chocolate that "accidentally" falls on his lips, he finally gives in to the temptation and devours more chocolate, before collapsing into tears of shame and delight. This is a classic example of the saint falling prey to his own inner sinner.

It must be noted that it is not just food that is a One's downfall; it can be illicit sex, drugs, theft, fraud, alcohol, or any number of other morally bad actions.

How They View their Bodies

Seeking perfection, Type Ones will feel that their bodies need to be perfect, in whatever way they choose to view perfection. For some Ones, this may take the form of "My body is my temple"; for others, it may mean an emphasis on being toned, having no cellulite, being super fit, or sticking stringently to a religious belief about food.

The body has base urges, or desires, and less integrated Ones believe that these must be quelled through discipline. The body is seen as the enemy—something that needs to be dominated. In order to gain the fitness/figure the One desires, there must be pain. It's an old-fashioned evangelical kind of viewpoint of "sins of the flesh." Should the One view their body as extremely imperfect, they may avoid swimming pools or gyms, where their "faulty" figures will be exposed.

Ones don't need outsiders to criticize their figures; they do a damn good job of it themselves! Too fat. Too thin. Boobs too small, large, or sagging. Butt too big. Thighs too dimpled… They will judge their figures harshly and inevitably find themselves lacking in some way. They may find themselves being critical of others' figures and approach to eating, but generally, they are even more critical of themselves.

Here, though, I need to touch on the Instinctual types as they relate to the One. Self-Preservation Ones would channel the need for perfection into themselves: to make themselves perfect. Social Ones would want to be role models in society: to stand above others. Sexual Ones would take the passion of perfectionism and focus it outward (counterphobic) into the world, thus desiring to perfect others. They may seem oblivious of their own bad eating habits, excess weight, or lack of exercise, yet hone in on other's failings.[1] Understandably then, they may be overweight and avoid seeing it.

Addictions

Ones are normally controlled and don't want to do the wrong thing, so obvious over-indulgence is not common. They tend to be sensible and disciplined. There are exceptions. I have interacted with a Type One who prided himself on the fact that he never touched a drop of alcohol, yet was blind to his addiction to unhealthy food, which left him very overweight.

When Ones disintegrate, they head toward hedonistic behavior and may binge-drink or get hooked on diets or diet pills.[2] They can become obsessive about weight loss and take whatever pills they can to improve their cause.

There can also be an aspect of denial to their addictions—imagine the teetotaler drinking cough mixture, or a woman I met once who drank herself into an early grave on certain healing tinctures that were formulated with alcohol. The tension of being "good" and doing the right thing needs release, and if it's not directed to say, sport, alcohol may be an option.

In organizations such as the Alcoholics Anonymous and its Twelve Step Program, Ones will feel comfortable with the imposed rules and get annoyed with others who are unable to implement them to the same degree. They may develop a self-righteous approach, being sober yet angry, unable to enjoy life or have fun, unless they do the inner emotional healing work required to truly heal. This rigidity could eventually reopen the doors to addiction.

Childhood

Ones learned that they got brownie points by being good and doing what was right, at the expense of what they really wanted. They were the children who ate the fruit at the birthday party, in lieu of the fudge and chocolate cake, because they knew that doing so would win them parental approval, rather than because they wanted the fruit.

As children, the message came across either directly or indirectly that they weren't good enough, imperfect in some way, particularly in relation to their biological needs. They may have had strictly religious parent(s) who judged their infantile needs as sinful. Their main protective figure may have been overtly strict or contrastingly, they may have lacked the support and guidance of this figure, so they developed their own set of guidelines, often more rigid than those they experienced in their childhoods.[3] Some Type Ones may have had little structure as children and so attempt to create rules and routines by which to live as compensation.

If the message they received when they were growing up was that it is bad to drink spirits, Type Ones may decide to not drink alcohol at all, to be even more beyond reproach. If the family value was to eat little meat, then becoming a vegan would see them rise even higher in their own personal judgment ranks. They may then feel obliged to "improve" the eating habits of those around them (remember the holier-than-thou vegan at the barbeque?).

Diets for Ones

Ones, as I've mentioned, are unlikely to be very overweight, although there are obviously exceptions. But while they may seem healthy, they still may have a less than healthy approach to eating and drinking.

The way for Ones to approach losing weight will be to use rules, precise weighing of food, and a regimented approach to dieting. Discipline and resolve are their strengths. Diet pills are also an attractive option.[2]

Fasting or detoxing also falls into the same category of withholding and discipline. Ones pride themselves on sublimating their desires, so not having the cake makes them feel good about themselves. Virtue is their reward, rather than necessarily wanting to lose weight. They are proud of their self-control and cannot understand the lack of it in others. It's easy to see why fasting would present the ultimate reward for both purification and abstinence.

While at healthier levels, fasting might be a spiritual practice to cleanse and revitalize the body, and this desire could be found in all types, fasting and fad dieting under stress, can translate as a punishment and desire for control, in a world where Ones feel they have somehow failed. Even the smallest indulgence, such as a sprinkling of sugar on a cup of green tea can cause panic, a feeling of being out of control and persistent self-criticism, which again gnaws at self-esteem.

Ones will stoically sit eating a meager or bland meal, believing that in doing so they are becoming better individuals. The pleasure of eating becomes a source of anxiety, however, as the One strives to adhere to a rigid diet. This can lead to eating extremely healthily in public and bingeing badly when alone. This is followed by massive self-recrimination and restrictions, which once again leads to the very tension that expresses itself through destructive eating.

Ones need to see that diets differ worldwide and that there are many different viewpoints as to what is the correct way to eat, and that theirs is not the only way. Understanding this allows Ones to see that there needs to be moderation in their self-imposed diet regime. They need to allow themselves to agree on the 80/20 principle, where 80 percent of the time they follow the eating plan and 20 percent of the time it's acceptable to deviate from it without self-recrimination. This is a far healthier mental approach.

To overcome any resistance to changing their eating behavior, if a One understands that through this change, they will gain more of what they want—perfection—they can be inspired to alter their approach.

If you're the dietitian, doctor, or therapist seeing a Type One, be aware that when you delve deeper into the unconscious of any type, the ego will resist and try to lead you away from the issue as a defense mechanism. If you're not aware of this, you may inadvertently take the bait and be prevented from doing the deeper work required to assist your patient.

As a result of their desire for perfectionism, Ones find criticism hard to absorb.[4] As a means of avoiding delving into the hidden places they experience as faults, they may embark on long, and often interesting stories, whilst avoiding the bigger issue that the problem is only a problem because of their perfectionistic fixation. As a therapist, you may get so drawn into these tales you miss the real work or issues that need to be addressed.[5]

Exercise

It's no surprise to learn that Ones adhere rigidly to their exercise routines. Should the routine be broken and self-recrimination set in, they may suddenly go from "hero to zero" activity, justifying it by saying, "If I can't do it all as stipulated, I'll do nothing." Ones enjoy discipline, so they usually work with a personal trainer or instructor to formulate their regime or rules of training. They do not, however, take kindly to advice from others, often seeing it as criticism. Because they view exercise as a "no pain, no gain" situation, it is seldom experienced as fun. In fact, they may see sport as frivolous and avoid it in favor of more "serious" pursuits. It's a means to reach a goal, which they often set unrealistically high and then feel they have failed when it's not attained.

As a result, whatever regime Ones follow may be repetitive and devoid of distraction, such as social interaction. As with eating habits, exercise may be seen to be a bland, repetitive, or even painful punishment. Yoga, for instance, may be popular with Ones, because it involves discipline, little personal interaction, and repetition, and the aim of perfecting yourself is appealing. Should the instructor, however, decide to deviate from the accepted routine, Ones may find this annoying ("She's not teaching yoga the proper way").

In team sports, they will be the member keeping the others in check. They will feel mortified if they think they have let the team down and can be equally harsh on others who they feel have not pulled their weight. Consequently, they may feel more attracted to solo sports where they will not let anyone down or be let down, such as marathon running and swimming.

They can be very hard on themselves when they perceive they have not lived up to their expectations. "If I say I'll go to the gym and then don't, it worries me the whole day. I get angry with myself for being so undisciplined, or if I do go, for not pushing myself more," Mike, a Type One, explained to me.

Ones can have idealistic desires for themselves, which in sport can manifest as a desire to leave their mark in some way: to be the sportsperson others look up to, to be the epitome of good sportsmanship and in so doing, to reform, inspire, and improve others. At Level 3 of the Nine Developmental Levels (with Level 1 being the healthiest and Level 9 the least healthy), the term used for this is The Level of Social Role.[6] (See Levels of Development – How Emotionally/Mentally Healthy You Are on page 22.)

At this level, you might find Type Ones in the role of teacher, where they not only practice the sport or exercise but pass on the knowledge to others, in order to demonstrate a desired path to remedy their health. Think of the yoga practitioner who becomes a yoga teacher, keen to instruct others and show them the right way to do the exercises.

Ones are ordered and so easily schedule a set time for exercise. Because it's seldom enjoyable, exercise becomes more a case of "I should," than

"Great, at last I can cycle." They push themselves hard and are unforgiving of their weaknesses.

As with eating, an 80 percent adherence to the sporting routine, combined with a 20 percent allowance for time off or relaxation would be a healthy option. Adding flexibility to a chosen sport could create much needed enjoyment.

How to Inspire Ones

For Ones starting a diet or exercise routine motivation is key, otherwise, they'll find themselves gradually slipping back into bad habits. So how would you as a Type One motivate yourself? It's simple, look at what you strive for in life. Most Ones want to reform the world, make it a better place. If through your actions you can inspire others to do the same, then you will feel a sense of achievement. Through your food choices and exercise regime, realize that what you are creating is a better you—more perfection, more integrity of being, and a role model for those seeking to better themselves as well. You're "walking the talk." When you find yourself slipping, remind yourself of these ideals and savor doing what is right for yourself.

Levels of Health
(See note on page 22)

Healthy

My father, a One, lived into his nineties and was always trim and healthy. He ate sensibly his entire life and swam regularly in the sea and in swimming pools. Even when he was over 90, he would get up at 6 a.m. to do so. I can still see him now, towel in hand, waiting for me to accompany him on an early-morning swim every weekday.

He also applied this discipline to his food choices. He would very occasionally allow himself a slice of delicious cake, and he did enjoy a glass or two of red wine, but I never saw him overindulge in food or alcohol in all the years I knew him. He simply did not understand why others needed to pile their plates high or eat fatty fast foods. In fact, I don't believe he ever ate a fast-food meal. It just did not attract him or fit into his inventory of what appealed to him.

A healthy One is far less judgmental of themselves and others. There is a nobleness and pureness about them. They truly do the right thing. Think of a sportsman who stops his race to help an injured competitor or, as I witnessed in a kite-boarding competition, one competitor take the board washed up onshore to a stranded competitor in his heat. They exhibit sportsmanship, and there is a nobleness and impeccable manner about their actions. They can see that their harsh criticism of others is, in effect, an attempt to quell their own repressed desires. As C. G. Jung so succinctly puts it in *Memories, Dreams, Reflections*:

> "But what if I should discover that the least among them all, the poorest of all the beggars, the most impudent of all the offenders, the very enemy himself—that these are within me, and that I myself stand in need of the alms of my own kindness—that I myself am the enemy who must be loved—what then?"

Healthy Ones allow themselves to enjoy life and have fun without the need for self-judgment.

Average

As Ones become less healthy emotionally, their self-criticism of their own or others' eating habits will escalate. They may become increasingly fussy about their food and how it's prepared. Fad eating may start to creep in, together with a moral superiority regarding their diet regime. Ever been with a vegetarian who believed that their diet would ensure their spiritual enlightenment while they looked disdainfully down their noses at all the non-vegetarians at the table?

I remember being told the story of an esteemed Buddhist monk who was visiting and teaching a group of his Western followers. They were all strictly vegetarian and so were horrified when, during their yoga class, the unmistakable smell of his boiled lamb came wafting through the temple. Growing up in the Himalayan Mountains, where crops are seldom able to grow, the monk's staple food was lamb. His teachings then came into question, simply because of his food choice.

It's not that vegetarianism is not a great and healthy way of life; it's just the moral superiority that Ones can overlay onto this and other preferred ways of eating can cause them problems with other more open-minded eaters. As noted earlier, as Ones disintegrate they can start to compulsively label foods as "good" or "bad" and becoming militant about applying the rules to themselves and enjoying the moral high ground this allows them.

I've observed Ones sigh reproachfully as others have a piece of chocolate, for instance, only to be found eating an entire slab surreptitiously.

In their efforts to eat healthily, Ones may overlook that the bland food they are eating may have hidden fats or calories. An example would be drinking a cup of ginger tea rather than regular black tea, not realizing that the packaged ginger tea sweetened with honey may, in fact, be loaded with sugary calories.

As they become less emotionally healthy, Ones begins to be more fanatical about wrong and right in many aspects of life, including food. Colleagues, friends, and family might find themselves being preached to in terms of what they should or should not eat or drink.

Unhealthy

Their approach to eating becomes more militant and rigid as Ones disintegrate, such as the vegetarian (I'm sure you've encountered a few) convinced that their way is the only way of living. They want to change eating patterns for the good of all and can become fanatical and judgmental in their views.

All those who in the minds of the One have got it wrong will be harshly criticized. Ones love perfection and find it hard to accept anything that is not in line with their understanding of perfection. If they decide that being a vegan is the right and proper thing to do, then they will find it hard not to judge a partner, colleague, or friend who happily munches their way through a steak. This frustration and resentment toward others for not adopting the One's stance can result in tirades (usually behind closed doors).

There is nothing more annoying than being about to tuck into a slice of black forest gateau only to have the One at the table say pointedly, "I thought you were trying to cut out sugar and wheat." A One may see that as constructive criticism; you may experience it as a hurtful and judgmental desire to spoil your enjoyment.

I remember an ice cream parlor called Sinnful Ice-cream, which spoke to the One's notion that enjoyment = sin. Ones are afraid that giving in to these delights will open up the potential for their instinctual or animalistic nature to take over.

Remember Stig, the minister in the Swedish film *As it is in Heaven*, who moralistically refuses to allow his sexual desires to be fulfilled in his relationship with his wife, only to be discovered reading pornographic magazines?

Given the rigidity in food choices that occurs as Ones start to become more disintegrated or unhealthy, it's understandable why so many sufferers of anorexia nervosa are found to have the Type One personality. This doesn't mean that less healthy Ones will suffer from this illness or that all anorexia sufferers are Ones, but the tendency is there.

Anorexics either have convinced themselves that they have no appetite or interest in food (the model picking at a lettuce leaf) in their pursuit of the perfect figure or they have convinced themselves that they need to lose weight and need to purge whatever they have consumed (bulimia). People who suffer from anorexia nervosa have not lost their appetite, but rather have restricted their food intake because of an irrational fear of gaining weight.

In keeping with the personality of a One, the anorexia nervosa sufferer is a perfectionist. When not meeting whatever target she has set herself (and often these can be unrealistic), her inner critic berates her for being out of control, so she looks for what she can control, which often becomes weight and food intake.

As a One starts to confront this black versus white ambiguity within themselves, and able to let go of the need to judge themselves and others, they can allow themselves the odd indulgence without recrimination. Moderation is the way to approach eating and drinking ("A little of what you fancy does you good…"), neither harshly restrictive nor wildly gluttonous, but able to appreciate the joy that well-prepared food can give.

Summary

Healthy, wise Ones see the goodness inherent in life as it is and impart nobility to the world in which they live. They let go of the need to judge their bodies as being wrong ("sins of the flesh" thinking), something that requires correction or punishment; rather, they experience the joy that is inherent in their physical selves.

Ones need to release the need to make everyone, themselves included, perfect and realize that beyond the divine perfection exists an acceptance of the way things are (and that includes the odd wobbly bit and pop tart). They can allow themselves to savor a great Chardonnay, indulge in the delights of a superbly prepared filet or a freshly baked, buttery croissant. No harm will come if enjoyed occasionally. Joy does not require perfection. Joy is the acceptance of what is, as it is. They need to feel that they are worthy of enjoyable, sensual experiences and that others' viewpoints on food and other matters are not threatening, but rather, an interesting alternative.

They judge neither themselves nor anyone else and have a truly impartial view of their world. This is perfection made real.

Type Two
The Giving Gorger or the Humble Helper

The Issue

Twos substitute a craving for intimacy with a craving for food. Eating becomes a way of trying to feed the heart. Unpleasant feelings of not being cared about result in comfort eating, hence the desire for sweet foods to replace the lack of life's sweetness.

Overview of Type Two

The term The Helper[1] or Giver accurately describes the warm personality (and wounding) of a Type Two. Twos need to be needed, and they create dependent needs in others by being extremely helpful and loving. As such, they are the most people-oriented of all the Enneagram types.

No gift is too large, no task too great, and no kind deed not doable for a helpful Two. They are the person who remembers your birthday and sends a card. Who never fails to produce your favorite dish and has it waiting for you when you visit. Who will drive across town to assist an elderly relative or help at the school concert. There is seemingly no end to their ability to give.

When healthy, they truly are the world's nurturers, able to lovingly care for themselves and others—the mothers of the world in archetypal form. Selfless and loving unconditionally, they strive to make the world a more loving and comfortable place for others. When healthy, they give with no expectation of getting. They are humble and give freely of their warm, nurturing nature. They are deeply compassionate, emotionally aware, and forgiving of the foibles of others. At a healthy level, many Twos have a healing effect simply by being present. There is no need to boost themselves to overcome the feeling that they are unworthy of being loved, as one can't help warming to them. They are usually good organizers and attuned to the needs of others. Affectionate and loving, they can work selflessly in service of others.

To understand a Type Two, think of the title of the Carole King hit song, "You've Got a Friend": Twos pride themselves on helping those in need.

But in average and unhealthy Twos, there is a hidden motivation other than kind generosity to their good deeds (of which they are often completely unaware). They crave intimacy and believe that love comes through doing things for others, that love has to be earned. They'll flatter, people-please, seduce, and can be very manipulative if they feel instinctively that it will create the warmth and relationships that are so important to them.

This need to be needed can lead to rescuer and martyr type behavior and seeking relationships where they can assume the role of savior or redeemer (and create co-dependencies). They can then start to believe that the people around them could not cope without them ("The place would fall apart if it wasn't for me"), hence the issue of pride that arises as their passion. Note: "Passion" here refers to the Enneagram and Biblical sense of being caught up in the spell of an issue or having a blind spot, not the more contemporary meaning of desire.

What Type Twos sometimes find hard to accept is that there is a "giving to get" agenda alongside their kind deeds. It's very important to them to be appreciated and to get the love they've been working so hard for. If they don't receive this appreciation, they can become angry and lash out. If you give them something, their dilemma becomes what to give you back. "After all I've done for you…" or "Fine. You go and enjoy yourself while I do the work…" would be common phrases that less healthy Twos might use.

As they become increasingly unhealthy, insincerity can arise. Boundaries are ignored. They can spread gossip, yet maintain a sanctimonious view of their behavior, as in "You need me…" and "I do so much for so many people." They become increasingly co-dependent and manipulative, blaming others for issues they have created, while simultaneously being terrified of being dumped by them.

But Twos who are prepared to work through their disintegration can achieve their rightful roles as altruistic, loving nurturers (both of themselves and the world). Generous, supporting, and encouraging, they assume a vital role in society.

Career Choices

You'll find Twos working for charities, as junior school teachers, in human resource departments, sales, working with the elderly, stay-at-home parents, the archetypal Jewish mother,[2] caterers, paramedics, or in the hospitality industry.

Eating Triggers

A common trigger for overeating in a Type Two is feelings of self-pity, loneliness, and lack of love. (*In spite of all I do for others, no one loves or appreciates me. Maybe I'm just not worthy of being loved. I'll feel better after I've had a packet of chocolate biscuits.*) Not feeling worthy of being loved is reinforced as a Two gains weight, resulting in more comfort eating, and so the spiral continues downward.

How Type Twos Approach Eating

When we were babies, the way we experienced love was through breast-feeding and our mother's nurturing. With a Two, when love is absent or removed, attempting to replace love with food becomes a very real option (love-starved = feeling physically starved). Kissing and eating are both oral experiences. So bingeing away (stuffing down) their feelings of being unloved and lonely is how Type Twos attempt to eat away at their gnawing feelings of lack of self-worth. Food becomes the emotional uplift they need when feeling lonely or unappreciated. This can vary from a simple sweet occasionally, to full-on binge eating, depending on the severity of the feelings.

"When life is not sweet, eating a sweet may help" is the unconscious message. As a result, they are drawn to the sweet things in life—chocolate, sweets, cakes, and carbohydrates (which turn into sugar in the body).

Twos Eating Out

Being people-oriented, Twos love to go out and socialize. They enjoy eating and people, so restaurant experiences are a way of nurturing themselves and others, which is essential for Twos. They can find it very hard if they find themselves in partnership with one of the more introverted types who don't enjoy socializing.

To imagine a Two entertaining, think of the typical Italian mother and her lovingly prepared meal served at a food-laden table to a host of family and friends, with much wine and laughter. Meals are sensuously enjoyed.

If a Two is invited to your house, they'll be the first in the kitchen after the meal to wash the dishes or stack the dishwasher. As such, they make great guests! Type Twos battle with boundary issues. They often can't resist taking over the kitchen, which some types will find a relief while others may find invasive. Don't be surprised if they reach across the table and take a taste from your plate, or invite you to do the same. For most people this may not be an issue, but for some it can be very annoying.

Twos are community minded, so if it's a church bazaar or a school fund-raiser, the Two will be out in front, tossing pancakes or putting dollops of cream onto the headmaster's waffle, while chatting to him in a relaxed, familiar (sometimes overly so) manner. Twos enjoy sharing food, so may order according to what they know their partner would like to share.

They are going to want to go to restaurants where the waiter knows them by name, they have a rapport with the chef, and can lavish delicious treats on their loved one(s).

Twos Entertaining at Home

As warm nurturers, Twos often enjoy cooking and/or baking. It's another way of demonstrating love and care. You will seldom leave the home of a Two hungry (you may even get to carry out the leftovers!). The Two will be there helping you to another slice of that divine cheesecake or insisting you have a second portion of their homemade stroganoff. Fiddly food won't work. Think big, hearty stews, comfort casseroles, and "kiss your thighs goodbye" desserts. Everyone is welcome. A friend from out of town? A visiting relation? No problem; just bring them along. They will likely prepare way too much food, rather than run the risk of being seen as not having enough to give.

My parents had a Two as a friend. Large and jolly, she always had sweets on hand, and we loved going to her home. Candy or cookies were kept in large jars for our small eyes to relish. The same applies for colleagues in the office, who may love Twos because of the drawer of treats they keep.

Twos are gregarious and warm, so entertaining is a natural expression of their warmth and generosity. They are great hosts/hostesses, genuinely interested in the dietary requirements of others, and remember likes and dislikes for the next visit. Comment on a favorite dish? Your helpful Two will remember and be sure to produce it the next time you're around.

Their homes often become the place for people to meet and enjoy a Two's generous, nurturing nature. Not always neat like a Type One's home, Type Twos view their abodes as demonstrations of loving warmth. Delicious baking smells, pets aplenty, indications of self-made crafts or your favorite drink poured especially for you are ways they demonstrate their caring. For many Type Twos food is love and they view preparing and sharing meals as an expression of love. They may overextend themselves in their attempts to please.

When Twos prepare food, the temptation for "tasting" along the way is always present, which can sabotage weight-loss programs! It's also important to prepare what a partner or others enjoy, rather than making what they would most like to eat. Following a diet becomes hard unless the partner buys into the eating plan as well; a Two will have more energy invested in eating like their partners than in doing their own thing and eating more healthily. (Of course, the opposite is true if the partner adopts a healthier eating plan.)

Twos with a One wing are known as The Servant in the Enneagram tradition of Riso / Hudson, and as The Hostess when they have a Three wing.[3] It's a subtle difference, but the One wing indicates that they enjoy waiting on others while the Three aspect has them enjoying shining in social circles as an amazing host/hostess.

The "giving to get" expectations of less healthy expressions of Twos can emerge in entertaining contexts, along the lines of thoughts such as *I've invited them twice to my house for supper, and they've never invited me back.*

Food Choices

Think of food as love. What food would most represent love to a Two? Food they ate when with a loved one, which could mean Mum's home-cooked meals, a special trifle enjoyed at family celebrations, the meal you ate together when you first met. All of these will nurture the Two, but bland and boring will not. They want the sensuous comfort food of chocolate soufflé as the liquid chocolate inside oozes out of the top, the buttery richness of a sage and burnt butter sauce on homemade pasta. Food = love, and love = comfort and intimacy.

As such, they may over-shop, buying more items than they could realistically consume, and be wooed by sensual smells and tantalizing packaging. You'll seldom find a Two's larder empty. They also will use gift buying as an excuse to shop, purchasing treats for themselves at the same time as buying gifts for others.

Because they are caring, loving people, some Type Twos may even become vegans or vegetarians, simply so as not to feel guilty about eating another sentient being. The idea of the cruelty that occurs to animals does not sit comfortably with them.

What You May Not See

The entire day, the Two has gone to a lot of trouble to prepare dinner. The family has arrived late and gulped food down before heading to the TV.

Just when you're feeling all love and kindness from the Two in your life, whoosh! This other person appears: over-sensitive or even openly angry. Days or even years of bottling up their hurt, frustration at not being appreciated, or feeling ignored explodes into potentially destructive action, threatening to ruin the relationships they have been working so hard to nurture. You may find that they have even kept a tally of all their kind deeds, which they perceive have not been reciprocated.

"I do all or at least 80 percent of the giving in my relationship," a Two confided to me. "It's just my nature. I get angry, though, when that isn't acknowledged." Twos need to be appreciated, so after that meal, be sure to send them a thank-you note (or better still, call them).

How They View Their Bodies

Type Twos are so focused on the needs of others they may totally ignore the needs of their own bodies, or at very least, view these needs in a lesser light. They may want to eat healthily, but their partner's need for fatty, fried foods may have them cooking this way, both to gain the appreciation of the partner and to be eating the same food together in a display of intimate eating interaction.

Everything and everyone is more important than the Two's needs which, like their appearance, they may downplay. Doing for others is more important than focusing on their appearance, and as long as their body is well enough to help or woo others, this is often sufficient for the Two. However, presenting a youthful, attractive appearance will help them get the intimacy they crave (if not in a relationship), and the seductive[4] role of looking good is important, particularly for Sexual Type Twos, the *femme fatales* of the Enneagram.[5] For women, this may mean wearing low-cut dresses with revealing slits up the side (think burlesque dancers); for men, it may mean donning skin-tight pants with an open neck shirt to reveal a well-exercised six-pack. Social Twos may power dress to appear impressive.

Twos often have soft features and voluptuous curves, so adding to the curves with overeating would enhance the "earth mother" or nurturer look. They often maintain their youthful looks longer than other types. This is particularly true for Self-Preservation Twos.[6]

Addictions

When doing for others doesn't create the desired intimate outcome, leaving them still attempting to get the love they crave, some less healthy Twos may become focused on their perceived health issues as a means of receiving the nurturing they desire. If they are emotionally unhealthy, some Twos may even develop illnesses (usually often not able to be cured or defined) to get the love and attention they have been trying to get by doing things for others.

This focus on personal health issues can lead unhealthy Twos to become addicted to over-the-counter medications,[7] such as strong painkillers for a sore back or headaches, for example. Too much sugar in coffee, sugary sodas, cakes, sweets—whatever offers the hope of sweetness in life will be attractive to an unhappy Two.

They may also be the classic enabler for others who have addictions, believing that through their "love" they will be able to save the loved one. If they themselves are addicts, then saving another person can be a way of avoiding doing the work to save themselves. Twos may leave one type of addict, only to find themselves with another in the next relationship.

Childhood

As a child, Twos soon come to understand that the love they seek needs to be earned rather than simply experienced unconditionally, so they begin to second-guess their carers/parents (What can I do for Mum that may reward me with what I need?). They fit easily into the role of "mother's little helper," where their needs are not as important as those of the parent/carer. This reads then as "I am only worthy of being loved if I am being loving toward others." The needs of the Two are suppressed and restricted and emerge as doing for others. When they don't get the love they so desire, this creates anger and confusion (How much more do I have to give to get what I need?).

When siblings who do little appear to receive more love, this creates confusion for the Two (*What more do I have to do to be loved?*). They start to become sensitive to what a parent (and later, others) may need

(*Mum's looking tired. I'll offer to make her tea*). This starts a lifetime habit of focusing on the needs of others while ignoring their own. Compounding the issue may be the strong religious belief that to focus on your own needs is selfish. So a child might want the last slice of cake but would rather get greater attention from praising parents by handing it over to another sibling.

Diets for Twos

When it comes to a Two following an eating plan, if they become stressed, they will not want to be seen to be nurturing themselves but rather need to frame it as being beneficial to others (If I am healthy, Sue won't need to worry about me or If I look good, then it will build Joe's self-esteem by having an attractive partner). Anything, in fact, that makes the program appear not to be a selfish endeavor but a kind and caring act for others.

While Twos may crave sweet treats and comfort foods, the guilt that follows (Type Twos, Threes, and Fours have issues with guilt and blame) may drive them in extreme cases to bulimia (*I binge to feel better and instead feel guilty and ashamed for doing so. To help eradicate these feelings, I may use laxatives, diuretics, enemas, force myself to vomit, or throw myself into an extreme exercise routine*). Whereas Type Ones are more likely to suffer from anorexia, where a significant weight loss is apparent, in order to look "perfect," a Type Two's motivation is to supress feelings of being unloved and unlovable through binge eating. People with bulimia most often maintain an average weight (or slightly above or below), which makes it harder to detect.

Most often this is triggered through weight-loss diets which, in the unconscious mind of a Type Two, equate to the withdrawal of love—Mum's breast removed, so to speak. This produces an overwhelming desire to experience nurturing/eating and to binge on whatever food is available, even if it's not appetizing. It's interesting that the choice often focuses on high sugar or high fat foods.[8] This is followed by guilt and the need to purge. And so the cycle continues, becoming more compulsive as it is repeated.

This leads to isolation (due to shame) and a fear of having a relationship that may expose the behavior, so Twos reject the very thing (love) they desire. Self-harming can also occur.

Naturally, very few Twos will be bulimic; it's just an extreme form of the potential desire for all that is sweet in life, when life holds little or no sweetness. If they understand the connection between feeling unappreciated and the warm, yummy feeling they feel when indulging in some sweet treat as a way of rewarding themselves (even if no one else is), Twos will be well on their way to working with their weight issues. True, unconditional love is not to be found in chocolate, despite what the media would have us believe!

Exercise

Twos may feel that exercise regimes only add to their feelings of being burdened, as the time taken to do them means less time to do all the things they are doing for others. Exercise may be intended but all too often is forgotten about in service to others. *(I just never get to the gym, I'm so busy helping at the community center. It's selfish to consider my exercise needs when others need genuine help.)* Through these and similar self-dialogues, Type Twos then can avoid exercise for the very best reasons. They do best when exercising with another person or as part of a team, where they feel they are helping the other succeed at a goal.

Much will depend on their significant other's needs or exercise routine ("If you want to work out, I'm there with you"). Even wanting to look good will not be seen as enhancing self-worth but enhancing the Two's worth to others (*If I look good, Pat will love me more*).

If the exercise routine can be seen to be enhancing the lives of others, then it has a far better chance of being regularly implemented (*I can't let Tom down. He needs me to help him stick to his workout routine*).

How to Inspire Twos

So what will motivate a Type Two to follow an exercise and / or eating plan? To be a source of love in the world, healthy Twos will need to demonstrate their ability to love and care for themselves first. The more they can experience their own cup as being full through their self-care, the more love they'll have to give others. Love then becomes an endless, limitless, flowing gift.

I've mentioned it earlier, but it will relate to being a more attractive and better "catch" or partner (*If I look better, I'll get more love*). This applies to all relationships, though, not just the role of loving partner. If I feel fulfilled and good about myself, then I can truly go the extra mile for all the people I interact with: I can remember the birthday of a friend, perform hidden acts of kindness, and give those I interact with the love and attention all humans desire.

Levels of Health

Healthy

Warm-hearted Twos have accepted that giving is not about getting; that they don't need to find comfort in unhealthy eating patterns; that empathy doesn't equate to losing yourself; that it's okay at times to be alone; that their needs are important and need to be met before they start giving to others; that they don't need the love of others to prove to themselves that they are lovable; and that love is unconditional. Feeling good about themselves allows them to encourage others to feel the same way about themselves. So encouragement and praise become genuine, rather than ingratiating flattery and pride is transformed into humility.

Average

As they become unhealthier, Twos feel they must do more to be loved, so they'll volunteer to organize the school bazaar, make food for the homeless, take in stray animals, or whatever it takes. Fearing that others may not want or like them, they increase their efforts to entertain, flatter, and please—anything to get closer to people. They may wine and dine others extravagantly, bake cakes for the new neighbors, or take meals to the sick, all of which is really kind and wonderful; it's just that the Two needs to be aware and honest with themselves regarding the true motivation for all they do. Only then can they let go of the need for prideful "the world can't do without me" feelings and work with the true reasons for their generosity.

Their enjoyment of being hosts/hostesses, waiting on others, tendency to extroversion and natural charm means they will try to create intimacy through shared eating. They have less self-control than many of the other types and so are more prone to snacking and tempting food choices, particularly if doing so brings them closer to others ("Let's be devils and open the Champagne, and I've got these amazing pretzels with cheese filling and your favorite chocolates…").

As they become increasingly needy, inevitably they drive away those they most want to be loved by.

Unhealthy

Unhealthy Twos continue blaming others for their weight ("I can't follow a diet/exercise regime because I'm too busy caring for your needs" or "I never have any time for myself").[9] For friends or partners, being made to feel guilty and suffocated with "love" creates the very opposite effect the

Two wants: people start leaving, as "loving care" is experienced as clingy, co-dependent, and manipulative behavior. They may also blame the dietitian or doctor for being incompetent, the diet itself for being flawed (even though they have cheated numerous times), those around them for "not supporting their efforts sufficiently," the food manufacturers, and just about anyone else, rather than accept responsibility themselves.

"I can't stand it," one woman said of her new boyfriend. "Every time I arrive home from work he's already there, fixing this, tinkering with that, preparing supper, watering the garden, painting the wall… It's exhausting because I'm expected to be grateful for what I never asked to be done in the first place. All I want is to relax quietly after work, and his neediness is such that I can't do that without being accused of being ungrateful."

The martyr and victim archetypes start to emerge in situations such as this ("No, you watch TV comfortably. I'm tired, but I'll wash the dishes and tidy up"). Creating dependencies may occur by, for instance, not allowing anyone else in the family to cook, so the family is dependent on the Two for their meals who at the same time is making everyone feel bad for not cooking. They believe that by worrying about your dietary needs, it will give them certain rights to your attention.

As people leave panic sets in, and the idea that they may have been "selfish" or in any way responsible is a concept they can't handle. They may lash out and blame others, inflate their good deeds, or even become ill (emotionally or physically) to finally get the attention they wanted all along.

Lonely, confused, and ashamed, they turn to the one thing that provides comfort—loads of sweet food!

When healthy, Twos order what they would like from the menu, and while cooking a nice meal for the family may be important, they bear their own needs in mind. They take time for their exercise routine, and sweetness comes from life itself, not sugary sweeteners. They learn to value themselves, their choices, and give themselves the love and nurturing they give others.

Summary

Twos need to learn to distinguish real intimacy from the intimacy they attempt to create from giving. As such, they need to give to themselves first, to fill their own cups before attempting to fill the cups of others. Being honest about the reason they put others first goes a long way toward bringing about true healing. When they work at self-improvement, be it through an eating plan, exercise routine, or seeing a therapist (or all three), they can truly move mountains.

Recognizing their warmth and friendliness as a strength, they can use this to work with and motivate both themselves and others to obtain a desired weight ("Let's meet every Tuesday and Friday at the gym, work out together for an hour, then we can have a smoothie afterwards"). This is a good way for a Two to maintain motivation, as they help themselves and others.

They need to create a loving relationship with themselves, first and foremost, so that they won't need to substitute the desire for love with food. Twos can be inspired to change if they understand that by doing so, they will feel better about themselves, leading to greater connection with others.

Type Three
Fast Food, Fast Life or the Chomping Champion

The Issue

Life is too hectic to worry about eating correctly as a Three's main focus is on goals and achievement, which may result in ignoring the body's needs. However, they may use their body and looks to enhance their status, so body image can be important.

Overview of Type Three

As their Riso/Hudson name Achiever or Helen Palmer's name The Performer suggest,[1] Threes are goal setting, image conscious, outwardly focused competitive types. They love to succeed, either as the "power behind the throne" or in their own shining spotlight. Known as the chameleons of the Enneagram, Threes will change their appearance and even the way they speak and act to suit the environment they are in. If a Three is running a successful business selling leather sandals they'll likely adopt a tie-dye, long-haired hippie look. Put them in a corporate setting, and they will be dressed for success in brand-name clothing and wearing an expensive watch.

Despite being one of the so-called "feeling" Enneagram types, Threes mask their true feelings under layers of efficient charm and diplomatic competency. They can talk equally to people from all walks of life. They have enormous drive and ambition and are keen to better themselves through all manner of interests, from art appreciatior to wine connoisseur.

They have a winning attitude and are adaptable to plans and projects. They work hard to achieve their goals and find it difficult to understand those less driven. They do not want to appear to have failed in any of the roles they assume, and find it hard to ask for guidance or help. When healthy, they become role models who inspire others to become the very best they can be.

Less healthy Threes, however, become increasingly desirous of recognition and may self-promote and exaggerate their accomplishments and ignoring or denying any failures. This need to can start leading to inauthentic behavior and the fear that they will be seen to be less amazing than they project. As a result, they may have problems with intimate relationships, fearing that others may see through the façade to the emptiness they feel inside. They can go from driving themselves to succeed to being utterly exhausted and shut down when no one can see them—Meryl Streep in the movie *The Devil Wears Prada* is a good example.

Unhealthy Threes have a fixation on deceit and will have no problem lying, scheming, sabotaging others, scapegoating, or claiming ownership of a successful project that was not theirs to claim, and hiding any traces of their failure or dishonest behavior. Healthy Threes, by contrast, work for the good of the world, are authentic, open, loving, modest, and inspiring to others.

Career Choices

Threes are highly efficient, so they do well in business, public relations, as personal assistant to a heavy-hitting boss, modeling, magazine work, politics, law, screen acting, pop music, marketing, advertising, fashion, motivational speaking, film making, life coaching, and areas involving networking. Corporate life suits many upwardly mobile Threes because they enjoy the skills required to climb the corporate ladder; in fact, anywhere where they will have a chance to shine and get the recognition and financial rewards they crave.

Eating Triggers

Stress, lack of time, and the need to eat-on-the-go may trigger junk food habits in Threes. Burnout and feelings of shame and perceived failure make them become like less healthy Nines, eating a lot of sugar-loaded foods or bad carbohydrates whilst vegging out for hours in front of the TV, until they recover sufficient confidence and self-belief to get back on track.

Be aware that you're heading into stress when you feel burnt out from overwork, opportunistic in your dealings with others, angry toward those close to you, and feeling something you may find hard to acknowledge—inner emptiness, where you're working hard to project an outer persona of success but you feel hollow and a failure inside.

How Threes Approach Eating

For a Three, eating can be another opportunity to display success. They enjoy having knowledge of food preparation techniques, as it adds to their status. Exotic or upmarket food choices allow them to come across as worldly wise—it's not so much about what they enjoy eating as what they enjoy telling others they have eaten. It's all about prestige, so whatever will enhance their image will be ordered or purchased.

In the pursuit of whatever goal they seek to accomplish, they can be disciplined and even talk themselves into believing that they don't like certain foods, or that eating is unimportant to them, just a means to an end. There is none of the emotional, comfort eating of a Type Two; rather, Threes are practical and can easily sever themselves from the instinctual food cravings of their bodies if it means reaching a goal.

Threes Eating Out

With Threes, eating out is likely to be at the trendiest/newest place in town. Even if their budget is limited, a salad at a top new restaurant will beat a three-course meal at Jo's Diner, because there you can see and be seen.

To improve their status, Threes may do courses on wine appreciation, so they don't let themselves down when they can't tell a Cabernet from a Shiraz. Or they may take an interest in cooking classes, top chefs or travel to improve their social skills. They love to share tips at the table on the best places to eat, the best wines to buy, the most effective diets, or the best ways to make money.

They are charming and good company in a group and are often popular as they create the ambiance for shyer, more introverted types. They enjoy listening to others to pick up information they can use with a similar group later on. "I even listen to things like helicopter pilots talking about the best helicopters—something I have no interest in as such, but I'm doing it for that future occasion when should I be with people who know about flying, I'll have information that's relevant to add to the conversation," a Type Three explained.

They may keep a list of the restaurants they want to visit. If it's in the Top 20 in the World restaurant list, then even better! Even if they are so broke they are living on fumes, Threes will be drawn to expensive restaurant experiences and choices. I knew a Three who would live on bread and lentils for most of the month, simply for the few nights when he could afford to dine out at the best restaurants, ordering top-class wines, and spending days afterwards reliving the event. Another Three friend of mine was having a hard time financially after a messy divorce, but she still insisted on taking 20 friends for a meal at one of the trendiest (most expensive) places in town on her birthday.

They may make menu choices based on what will look the best in a particular group of people. If it's vegetarians, they'll order even stricter vegan; if it's a business lunch with everyone else ordering steak, even if they do not enjoy steak, steak it will be. They want to make the best possible choice to impress the group they are with.

While they may be happy drinking the same healthy "green" shake every day, when eating out they would never order the same dish twice at the same restaurant. Even going to the same restaurant twice could make them tetchy. "I keep a list of restaurants on my phone so that I don't have to go to the same place twice. If people ask me about a restaurant, I want to be able to say I've been there," a Type Three remarked.

Power (business) breakfasts are likely to be very popular with a Three!

Threes Entertaining At Home

Threes may be more inclined to entertain at trendy restaurants than make a meal at home, but if in their constant need to better themselves being an expert cook becomes part of the agenda, they will pull out all the stops to impress others. With their need for efficiency and to feel of value, they will do their utmost to make the evening a lavish success. Budgets will be blown, mundane food excluded from the menu, and cheap wine tossed out in favor of what's perceived as being top of the range, as they strive to impress.

Even if they have never cooked a meal before, a Three will strive to "fake it until they make it." Meaning the local curry house may actually have prepared the meal, but a nifty transfer into their own casserole dish will make it appear as if it's just emerged from the Three's own oven. Or they may study recipes on YouTube the night before that look fantastic but are in fact relatively easy to prepare. They are going for that wow factor, which will lead others to heap praise and admiration onto their plates.

Their homes or apartments will need to reflect their success. Art by trendy new-name artists, unusual décor pieces of furniture, designer kitchenware, photos or trophies displaying their accomplishments, from skiing in Switzerland and climbing Mount Kilimanjaro to meeting the President or traveling on a luxury liner with famous friends, and certificates showing successful completion of courses, awards, diplomas, medals, degrees—well, you get the picture.[2] If they do not entertain, then they will invest that money in an upmarket car or trips abroad and keep their living space, clean, practical, and uncluttered.

Supper clubs will be popular with a Three as a way to mingle with others and possibly mix work and pleasure. Plus, if held at restaurants, it's a great way to visit the latest establishments.

Threes are charming and gracious hosts/hostesses. As noted earlier, they are chameleon-like and will alter the setting, meal, or clothes to make for an evening best suited to the types of people they are entertaining. If it's the trendy film crew set, they'll serve tasty canapes with cocktails. If its management from work, they'll just as easily produce perfectly cooked Beef Wellington as part of a five-course dinner. For friends, they'll appear to have "thrown together" a Tex-Mex buffet with mini margarita ice pops.

Sexual Threes tend to be the power behind the throne, supporting others in their success. As a Sexual Three, they will create the perfect ambiance for their significant other to shine, rather than the other two instinctual Three types where they will be more the focus. As the wife of a business man or important figure, they'll go out of their way to show off their home and partner in the best light to fast-track their partner's success.

To fail is not an option. They want to be outstanding in all they do and produce. Think of the mother who burns her batch of cookies destined for the bake sale and then buys some from the store and whacks them around a bit to make them appear homemade. That way she gives the appearance of being a baker, nearly as perfect as the store.

Alone, though, a Type Three may happily opt for leftovers or takeout.

Food Choices

Threes, as we know, enjoy improving themselves. Having greater insight into food and its preparation or better still, being on first-name terms with the farmer or producer, will enhance their social status. You get street credibility for knowing where the best place in town for sushi is or where the best cocktails can be obtained or how something is prepared—the more exotic the better! For instance, at a restaurant last night, a Type Three (who ironically is a vegetarian) was demonstrating to the rest of us how to tell how well done a steak is by pressing her hand to indicate doneness.

Choosing trendy food is a chance to make an upwardly mobile statement to others in the group. If those food options are not available (as in a menu featuring only common burgers or pizzas), or if they are eating alone without anyone to impress, food can simply be an uninteresting necessity. Type Threes can transfer their competitive nature and need for accreditation and success to the foods they eat. Two dishes that appear the same? The more expensive one must be better. Branded or unbranded? If it's on view, branded will always win. They are very aware of the best brand to purchase. Food becomes a way of displaying status.

"I'm so successful I can eat out at _____ restaurant."

"Others may think French champagne and Tanqueray gin are exotic, but I wouldn't order them because it's too cliché. I want to appear like I am knowledgeable about interesting gin and would order Bloedlemoen, Triple Three, or something else more unusual. I want people to be impressed—not that I can afford it so much as that I have good or unusual taste."

"My choice would be 80 percent pure cocoa, hand-crafted chocolate."

Food porn, or the habit of posting photos of your meal onto social media like Instagram, is a great way of displaying your success. "Hey guys, while you eat your grotty takeout, check out what I'm eating: Foie Gras Bourguignon at Ritzy's!" It's more about having an opinion about certain foods and drinks than wanting to show off as such. You want to appear sophisticated and worldly.

Because health is an internal issue, for the most part it doesn't overly concern Threes. As a result of rushing to get a job done or traveling frequently, they may make poor food choices—grabbing lunch on the run from fast-food joints, drinking a protein shake, picking up a few nutrition bars from the gas station, not eating or eating whatever they can find at home, from crackers to leftover pizza while working in front of a laptop. Coffee, black tea, caffeinated drinks, or anything that allows the Three to work longer hours will be attractive.

When they are not preparing food for others or needing to impress, they'll approach shopping in the organized, efficient, and practical manner that defines them. Daily food choices are not a big deal. They'll happily eat fried egg on toast every day and go big when eating out. Because they are social bunnies, their monthly restaurant bills often exceed their weekly grocery bills.

What You May Not See

Because Threes need to present an image of success and accomplishment, even though, deep down, they may feel emotionally vulnerable and perhaps worthless, they seldom ask for help or support. (Successful people are self-supporting. If I need help, then I'm not projecting achievement). Few people thus see the isolated, needy emptiness that many Threes feel. Because female Threes are usually successful and project confidence, men can find them threatening. Consequently, a Three woman, however beautiful and accomplished, may be alone. They are desired but seem unobtainable, so they convince themselves that this is the way they want to be (Partners are just a complicated hassle).

Threes have an ability to get the job done and put on hold their own feelings and emotions ("Even if someone says something really mean to me at work, I'll laugh it off and carry on with the task. Later, at home, I may cry about it, but chances are I'll have moved onto another activity by then, so I never have to feel the hurt").

To others, who don't see the vulnerable side as well as the shame of Threes, they can appear to be hard and unfeeling. At work, they feel safe and admired so working late becomes preferable to going home to an empty apartment or a partner who is angry and feeling estranged because they're working so hard.

A Type Three, Annette, described one of her typical Three dreams to me: "I was climbing a ladder to fix a hole in the ceiling. Everything was going well until I looked down and saw that instead of the floor there was this empty hole."

Burnout is a very real threat for Threes as they push themselves beyond their limits. Like unhealthy Nines, they can procrastinate and become unreliable—the very opposite of the polished image they like to project.

How They View Their Bodies

I remember a Three telling me that if she went to a party and was not the best dressed, most beautiful and admired woman there, she would leave. The statement amazed me (also the realization that with that viewpoint, I'd have missed many a great party!).

Success usually denotes success in all fields—supermom, superdad, supersportperson, superworker, and so forth. In some Threes, the body is a way of displaying their achievements. It's important to look the part, which is why cosmetic surgery is so popular. If you can't fake the cleavage, just make it with an insert here and a nip and tuck there.

As the numbers of Three women increase in the USA, so too does the surge in plastic surgery (previously, most Threes were men). In 2015 alone, statistics reveal that roughly one procedure was performed per

16 adults—1.7 million[3] cosmetic procedures in total. From 2000 to 2015, the number of cosmetic procedures jumped 115 percent! Buttock implants were the fastest-growing treatment. Men also got on the bandwagon, accounting for 40 percent of breast reduction procedures.[4]

The website *RealSelf* surveyed 700 people who had contacted a doctor for advice about cosmetic surgery. Part of the survey required them picking an adjective to describe why they wanted to have the procedure—76 percent chose "confidence." [5]

To enhance this desire for confidence, acceptance, and validation, clothes and accessories become another status symbol. The Gucci bag, the Vuitton top, the latest iPad—all will seem like "must haves" to the Three.

Some Threes seek status via their bodies, others through work, and some go after financial assets. Those whose focus is their bodies and its appeal can become "trophy brides," perfectly sculptured gym bunnies or dazzling toy-boys, who spend a lot of time creating the perfect look. I often see a man in the gym looking repeatedly into the mirror. He has obviously worked very hard to achieve his rippled body. He puts his baseball cap on one way, then moves it around to a different look, changing it again, all while flexing his muscles and devising the most appealing combination.

The trouble with needing the body to present success is that whilst perfect weight might be achieved, the perfect image changes according to fashion dictates, so it can remain an elusive goal. In truth, it's not the look that is the goal; subconsciously, it's the need to feel of value and to be validated, which seems to constantly slip through their manicured fingers. Even though they may have achieved the desired weight goal, if they aren't being admired the achievement feels empty.

If they are not getting accolades from their bodies, they may attempt to emotionally detach from them, seeing their bodies as an inanimate object. As such, the body's instinctual needs are ignored or avoided.

Addictions

Attempting to be up when feeling inwardly down requires a chemical boost, so as noted earlier, coffee, caffeine drinks, sugar, amphetamines,[6] stimulants, performance drugs (to win at all costs and enhance training intensity), ephedrine, cocaine, or steroids will be how Threes keep going. The down side, when the body collapses in exhaustion or the drugs start wearing off, is where they may deceive themselves as to the level of their addiction (I can quit whenever I want).

They will also start making up whatever stories they can to mask their deterioration. Think of famous sportspeople who spend years denying their drug usage before being inevitably caught. The need to achieve means that there is a huge potential for being attracted to performance-enhancing drugs. This need to win at all costs can also lead to bribery in sport, as we've witnessed in soccer, cricket, and point-shaving in college basketball for example.

Even in drug rehab programs, Threes will be attempting to prove to others how much more successful they are on the program. They will be the star rehab success story, even while avoiding the reasons they started taking drugs or alcohol in the first place. When the gap between the reality of the emptiness they feel and the image they need to project becomes too big, addictions and their effects create the fantasy that offers an escape from reality. Stimulants of any sort allow them to feel great and avoid tiredness, so they can work or work out longer and feel on top of the world.

Childhood

We live in an age where many children are told they can achieve whatever they desire, that there are no limits, bar the limitations of their dreams. They often leave school believing that a managerial position should be theirs within months of starting work, and have an inflated sense of self that we as parents have created, a world where children are often treated as mini gods and goddesses.

This is the Age of the Selfie, where it's all about the self—not the inner selfless self but the outer glitzy self. It's an age of wannabe Threes— where we believe that people really want to see endless images of ourselves on social media; where the number of "likes" on Facebook can build or break a person's sense of self; where we endlessly want to post our achievements in the hope that others will recognize and acknowledge the greatness we don't feel.

We are essentially in an age of Three thinking. Remember the book *Battle Hymn of the Tiger Mother* by Amy Chua? It's a good example of a Type Three mother pushing her children, often to draconian lengths, to succeed in many areas of life. The new breed of teenagers and young adults, the 20–30-year-olds, known as Millennials, Generation Y, or Generation

WE, are viewed as being anything from self-obsessed narcissists to open-minded and expressive.

According to the National Institutes of Health in the USA, Narcissistic Personality Disorder is three times higher in this generation than in the 65+ age group.[7] The increase in narcissistic personality disorder is alarming in a youth that is becoming obsessed with fame, doesn't believe in the need to work hard to achieve, and believes in landing top jobs straight out of college. Narcissistic personality disorder shows up in an inflated sense of self, in which sufferers believe that unlimited success, brilliance, and adoration (which they frame as love) is their right. They cannot deal with criticism, and spend much time fantasizing about their success, rather than actually working toward it. Social media obsession has been strongly linked to the increase of this disorder. It's not that all of this generation are Threes, but rather, that some of the aspects of this generation resemble a disintegrated Type Three.

Threes wanted to fulfill the subconscious expectation of their primary nurturing figure. For example, a Type Three woman I know holds a black belt in karate, was head girl, is a lifesaver, was the top student in her college, excelled at work... the list goes on. Threes feel that as children they were valued more for what they did than simply for being themselves. They are the heroes in the family, the stars at work, or the golden child in their society.[8]

They excel where the family failed. In some cases, they may attempt to compensate for the father (or main paternal figure) in the eyes of the mother (or main maternal figure). The only child who made it to university. The adult who was fast-tracked at work or who made bundles of cash while the rest of the siblings remained poor and less educated. They may be the athlete who achieved what their athletically minded parents did not. The actress who rose to achieve the kind of fame her mother had only dreamed of. The downside of this is they can never be average. Second simply is not an option. It's an uncomfortable place to be.

As a hero, you can't be wounded, so Threes may hide their wounds and loneliness under a façade of success (*I'm fabulous! Life is great! I'm a winner! I'm so sorted!*).

Diets for Threes

Threes love goals. Having a weight goal and then striving toward it is familiar territory for them. They'll have charts, self-help diet books, and goalplans—whatever it takes to track their weight-loss success.

When success at all costs is your mantra, a starvation diet may appear to be the solution, if the Three feels it will enhance their progress toward a desired goal—a good partner, a better position, more work, or simply being the best-looking person in the room. To this end, they'll buy the books, subscribe to the plans, or pay oodles of cash for products that will help them achieve their weight loss faster.

They are good at using visualization techniques to help achieve their dietary goals and, unlike Twos, can resist sugary temptations. They are self-starters and can motivate themselves into dietary action.

They may also ride on their past achievements in order to justify their current refusal to change unhealthy eating patterns, such as "I got to be Miss California 20 years ago, drinking martinis and eating burgers, so I don't see the need to change. It works for me." Even when diabetes may be looming, blood pressure is soaring, and cholesterol is way too high, if the outer appearance looks good, they will be hard to persuade to eat a healthier diet.

When the body becomes THE work goal, anorexia can arise. Not for perfection as with a Type One, but for supreme desirability so that they can get the strokes they seek.

Naturally, anyone with wounding that lies in achieving is going to hate to fail. If the diet isn't working they'll bail, citing other reasons for doing so (work pressures, burnout, and so on). They hope that this new avenue will provide a greater reward high.

Exercise

Because they view their body as the outer projection of success, appearance-oriented Threes may work out to the point of exhaustion. As in all other things in life, they may push themselves way too hard, then like the Type Nine their point of stretch, they may collapse in a heap and veg out in front of the TV with takeout for a weekend, not getting out of their pajamas.

Combine this ability to push themselves to the limit with a competitive nature, and they'll have a "win at all costs" approach. For some Threes, though, it's not all about winning. It's more about being acknowledged, as in, "There's Joe. He won the triathlon three times in a row."

Once set on a weight goal, though, the typical Three will, as they are inclined to do, throw everything at getting to their desired weight. They'll employ personal trainers, dietitians, coaches, whatever it takes, to get to the top of their game. They enjoy competition and so are attracted to sports such as marathons, triathlons, swimming, and running.

The body can become a way of achieving recognition, so, as noted earlier, cosmetic surgery may become a means to create a look that exercise can't. Tuck here, lift there, change the nose, enlarge the breasts—whatever will get them the admiration they desire.

Quick-fix solutions may be appealing and disregarded when they are perceived to be not fast enough in getting the result. Threes may cut corners, hoping that they'll still get the result with less time input. Expensive cosmetic creams and the like may appeal to them as a way to further enhance their looks and eradicate "flaws."

Bigorexia (formally known as muscle dysmorphia) is a disorder that can be common among Type Three men. The opposite of anorexia, where the person wants to be small, bigorexia (purported to be an issue with 10 percent of men in UK gyms and up to 54 percent of men in general)[9] is the desire is to create a bigger body (bigger as in more muscular). Wikipedia reports that the disorder is most prevalent in China, South Africa, and Latin America.

Bigorexia is an anxiety disorder often found in those who were teased or bullied, who feel small despite being strong and muscular. No amount of packing pectorals or sexy six-packs is ever enough to create the feeling of strength they desire. With the desire can come the abuse of anabolic steroids, protein shakes, and supplements. Family or work can suffer, as ever-increasing time needs to be spent at the gym. As the perceived gap grows between the body they believe they need and the body they believe they have, depression and suicidal thoughts may emerge.

Winning is not as important to Threes as the praise and accolades from winning are. If they are very overweight, going to the gym will be a grim mirror of their failure to maintain a good body. So they may avoid gyms altogether and opt for working out at home or with a private coach (or go back to working ridiculous hours and let go of the get-fit goal). If the goal is not being achieved by exercise, rather than experience failure they may throw themselves back into work or some other activity, then use this as the reason for the lack of achievement.

It's also important which gym a Three goes to. One Three told me: "I joke about it, but it is also true. I have the option of going to two gyms. Gym A is a much nicer and cleaner gym but gym B is the one I go to. Why? Because there are fewer attractive people there. No good-looking guys to feel shy in front of, no skinny girls to compare myself to, but now that I'm getting more toned, I am spending more time at gym A. I want to be seen and admired."

How to Inspire Threes

Getting Threes to set goals is easy—it's something they enjoy and are familiar with doing. Being successful with a diet or exercise program is yet another opportunity to be a star. If they understand that achieving their goal will result in enhancing their status, you'll have them on board. They will feel more valuable, more accomplished and more accepted [10]—examples and inspiration to others who want to become healthier and fitter.

Levels of Health

Healthy

When emotionally healthy, Type Threes will have their work/life well balanced. They are modest about their achievements, self-accepting and truthful. They no longer sell their souls to be validated by others and realize that self-worth is not about doing, but rather about being. They feel of value, not winning, shining, or being the hero, but just by showing up as themselves. The time spent seeking approval can now be spent validating others and becoming true role models, worthwhile and valuable members of society, rather than inflated balloons.

Average

As they become less emotionally healthy, work/life becomes increasingly unbalanced. They will have focused their achievement goals on gaining wealth and/or climbing the corporate ladder and valued their waistlines and health less, unless looking good is perceived to be an essential part of their career (for instance if they are a TV presenter, actor, or model). They start to spend more time enhancing themselves in the eyes of others. They want others to see how successful they are, and will work at enhancing that image at whatever cost to themselves. "All the world's a stage, and all the men and women merely players," wrote Shakespeare in *As You Like It*. For the Three, life is a stage on which they seek to find a way to take the lead role.

The desire for praise and acknowledgment can make them highly susceptible to manipulation by those seeking power over them, such as a partners, parents, or managers. Keep withholding the validation, and they'll keep trying harder to get it, which keeps the other person pulling the strings.

In their attempts to receive recognition and acceptance, they may follow a career path not necessarily of their choosing[11] but which they feel would be the choice of a parent, manager, or partner and offer the most potential for praise. They want the cleverest kids, the most stylish home, the best-looking partner, and to be the best at their sport, computer game, bed the largest number of partners, and so on. The desire to win can take several forms. In time, they can become detached from what they really enjoy and desire.

But they need quick-fix solutions, so they will indulge in diet drinks, frequent colonic therapies, steroids, or corrective surgery, all of which focus on their physical exterior while having little concern for the interior damage they might be causing. Remember many years back that women took pills containing tapeworms? They didn't care that the worms were slowly starving them of vital nutrients; they just wanted to be insta-thin!

Unhealthy

The particular form in which an unhealthy Three's woundedness comes out is in deceit—not necessarily telling lies but representing themselves to others in ways that are not an authentic reflection of who they are but that allows them to seem to be the best and win approval. In doing so they lie to themselves about feeling inadequate or lacking, favoring the ego self over the authentic soul self. What's left is an empty (but attractive) shell. They may cheat in the race, take banned substances—it doesn't matter as long as they can shine.

They head toward narcissism and want to show off their achievements to others. No matter the form it takes, they need to be the important star. To this end, they may view themselves as an object to be promoted, paraded, adorned, starved into beauty, using their attractiveness to seduce others into giving them what they desire—whatever it takes to reach their goal(s).

The next stage is often complete burnout, anger, hostility, and depression.

Threes when they move toward becoming healthy, have genuine self-worth, they value both their inner and outer selves, taking care of both.

The need to climb perceived winning ladders is replaced by being present with what is. The need to impress is gone and sees them using their many gifts to create organizations and structures that will benefit others. They order from the menu of life what will genuinely serve them best.

Summary

The good news for Type Threes is that, of all the types, if they set their mind to it they are most likely to succeed in their weight-loss goal. If the pressures of work or child rearing and juggling a career have had them packing on the pounds with fast food and bad food choices, if they prioritize weight loss they'll most likely stick to it. Most important, though, is to do it for themselves, so that they feel better about who they are (self-accepting) and are not motivated by the desire for approval of others. Doing inner work to connect with the lost side of themselves would be hugely beneficial. To this end a creative outlet, such as painting, pottery, gardening, journal writing, and so forth, would help them to connect their inner and outer worlds—and explore what is their true life's purpose—what inspires them.

Try being with yourself rather than doing. It will be a tough challenge, but it is the road home to your authentic self. Get inspired to change by realizing that here is an opportunity to achieve more—to present a better aspect of your goal and to embrace the success this offers. Being is as important as doing.

Type Four
Moody Muncher or Creative Connoisseur

The Issue

Mood and the focus on feelings determine the food choices of a Type Four. Food choices reflect how they feel. If sad, they'll comfort-eat; if they are feeling upbeat, they'll eat well.

Less integrated Fours sometimes feel a sense of entitlement in life; it's a counter to feelings of shame and a sense of lack within them *(If I feel lacking within, then surely what lies outside of me is the solution. My suffering gives me the right to demand what I need; yet when I get this object of my desire, it doesn't fulfill me long term)*. Much of a Four's experience involves enviously longing for what they feel they don't have.

If they fantasize about food that they desire, then they feel they deserve to eat it. Yet, even in obtaining what they desire, what they really desire seems always to elude them, so they conclude that the object of their desire is clearly what's at fault. Depression and feelings of insignificance can drive Fours into binges as a way to feel better. If they feel down and heavy, then bad food choices will mirror their dark feelings, just as healthier food reflects their healthier mind state.

Overview of Type Four

Anais Nin's quote sums up a Four's perspective on life: "Ordinary life does not interest me." Fours have a love of beauty and are introspective, individualistic, sensitive, intuitive, artistic, self-expressive, and often romantic. They are creative thinkers who enjoy pushing the boundaries of expected thinking.

When integrated, Fours are original, sensitive, gentle, and self-aware. This awareness means they have an intimate relationship with themselves and when outwardly focused, an intuitive understanding of the emotional pain others may be suffering. However, as they become less healthy, this awareness can turn into self-absorption.

They long for the buzz of intimate connection with others. "Will you walk into the fire with me?" they metaphorically ask.

If you see someone with a pink streak in their hair, covered in "dark" tattoos (skulls, snakes, fantasy, and so forth), with numerous piercings, dressed in vintage clothing, or wearing a flower in their hair, chances are you're looking at a Four.

The hipster[1] movement is a movement of Type Fours, although typically a hipster would not want to be identified as such, because then they would not feel unique. (Wikipedia describes the modern hipster movement thus: "It is broadly associated with indie and alternative music, a varied non-mainstream fashion sensibility, vintage and thrift-store-bought clothing, generally progressive political views, organic and artisanal foods, and *alternative* lifestyles.")

A deep feeling of shame creates the need to see themselves as different—above the rules of society. They want to be anything but boring, and they enjoy showing the world how different they are from others. (Ironically, when less healthy, a Four's self-absorption can make them appear boring to others.) They typically over-identify with their feelings, which makes them the most emotionally aware and expressive of all the types.

They commonly see themselves as being defective in some way and experience themselves as somehow being less fortunate than others, as if they drew the short straw in life, which leads them to feel envy toward people whose lives appear infinitely better. A common feeling expressed by Fours is that they feel as if they don't belong in the family they grew up with—as if their "real" family is somewhere else. Life itself can feel like a tragedy of sorts, in which they play the lead role. As the tragic actress/actor, they find meaning in their melancholy. They are comfortable with feeling melancholic, as if through this feeling they can experience the world with greater depth.

They can be emotionally dramatic and temperamental, demanding attention from others through their behavior. When not getting their needs met, they can become dismissive and critical of others, who they may see as mundane and superficial. When unhealthy, the creativity that flowed naturally becomes stuck, such as the best-selling writer who cannot find their mojo again. Filled with shame and self-loathing, they may lash out at others. Depression is common at this level, as well as seeing themselves as tragic victims (supposedly) tormented by the actions of others.

But should they choose to, Fours have the potential to move into being spontaneous, authentic, highly creative, self-aware beings.

Career Choices

Fours are the archetypal artists of the world, which is why they are most often involved in music, ballet, art, writing, poetry, interior design, animation, art direction, architecture, and so on. Even if not creating themselves, they are usually involved in creative fields, such as being an art critic or film editing. The other popular Type Four option is to be in the healing field, particularly the alternative healing world, and may work as reiki practitioners, yoga teachers, or more conventionally, psychologists or counselors.

Eating Triggers

Eating triggers take one of two forms:

1. Feeling themselves as defective in some way and having experienced themselves as somehow being less fortunate than others, creates a search for identity, which can manifest as choosing certain foods to enhance the current identity. ("I am a very spiritual person, so I don't eat meat." "I only drink Bordeaux wines.")

2. If they feel uncreative, ashamed, unstimulated, rejecting themselves, or worse still, boring, they may become slothful and withdraw into Type Two eating behavior, attempting to comfort eat to replace love.

When Fours are heading into areas where they feel stressed, it can show up as feelings of disassociation from others, hopelessness, co-dependency, and possibly depression. They can become quick to anger—from the outside, often being highly critical of others and apparently overlooking their own faults but, on the inside, have deep feelings of shame and self-loathing that are being projected onto those close to them. They may reject help, so getting them to see a therapist, dietitian, or other practitioner may be contemptuously disregarded. Eating provides a release.

How Fours Approach Eating

For a Four, food is another way of expressing their desired individuality. A Four who is an artist said: "I knew we could not really afford to buy food from the upmarket deli, but I find it fresher and better presented than the supermarket. Because I eat mostly salad and only certain meat cuts, that extra clean and fresh presentation is more important to me than budgetary restraints, so I buy my food there. The rest of the family eat mostly from the supermarket. It doesn't seem to be such a concern to them."

Eating becomes a way to express their uniqueness. So you'll find them as vegetarians with a gluten-intolerance who love chocolate—but only if 80 percent pure cocoa from Trinidad or some such country, and it must be fair trade—or organic-only eaters who eat free-range chickens and only drink certain types of coffee. Food needs to communicate their feelings, so a crisp, organic salad with unusual extras, such as pomegranate seeds, for example, shows others that they are light, aware, earth-conscious, yet tasteful and exotic. Consequently, they can be very particular (and even picky) in their food choices.

The exception would be if they are more unhealthy, in which case in focusing on their feelings they may lose contact with their hunger needs and nibble on junk food or whatever is easily available.

They can overly identify with the food they eat, so that if they weaken and eat "banned" food, they don't just feel guilt and remorse over the food they have eaten but feel bad about themselves, in general. If they eat foods they perceive as being "good," they then feel good and acceptable. "If I eat a roll for instance," a Four recounted, "I feel bloated afterwards and angry with myself for having messed up, when I knew this would be the result. It's almost like an extreme self-dislike related to what I've put in my body, which I see as being my temple."

The title of the book by Dr. Gillian McKeith, *You Are What You Eat: If Your Body Could Talk, What Would It Say About You?* sums up the Four's understanding of what they put into their bodies as reflecting their feelings.

Fours Eating Out

Restaurant choice is important for a Four. They would die rather than be seen at a chain restaurant that serves production line food slapped onto a plate and where quantity rules over quality. So "two for the price of one" burgers will not be enough to entice them in to dine, but the Wagyu burger on toasted sweet potato with homemade beetroot pickle will. They will read Eat Out, Foodism, Gourmet, or Bon Appetit and local fine dining magazines to find the newest restaurants and read online restaurant reviews without fail, then head to where the most exquisite food can be found.

Presented with a menu, a Four will be more likely to decide based on what they don't like eating rather than what they do.

An art director Four explained to me: "I don't eat chicken—I don't like the way they are reared—so I cancel those items, then I only like sirloin steak, not rump or filet, and possibly lamb, depending on the cut, so any other meat types I ignore. Anything with wheat or cheese, other than Parmesan or Feta, I'll discard, and I'm not wild about cooked vegetables. Once I've eliminated all those items, there is usually only a choice of one or two dishes to choose from, which makes things easy."

Fours use food to express their uniqueness so mundane chicken pot pie or burger and fries won't work, unless it will stand out in the group as being retro and quaintly old-fashioned, or the "burgers" are made from hand-reared lamb and the "fries" from sweet potato accompanied by a ripple of homemade whole grain mustard. I worked with a copywriter Four who would blow his whole eating out budget on a single night of fine dining and the very best wines, rather than lessen his taste with more frequent economic choices.

Just as with their choice of clothes, cars, décor, and so forth, Fours use food to enhance the belief that they are in some way special or unique—refined connoisseurs, particularly "aristocratic" Fours. (The wings create two types of Fours—Aristocrats, who have a Three wing, and Bohemians,[2] who have a Five wing. They act as the names imply.)

Fours have very strong opinions and aren't afraid to voice them. Even if they've never cooked a meal in their lives, they will be quick to point out with authority that there is too much cardamom or too little salt.

They love it when the barista remembers the exact way they enjoy their cappuccino. If the owner at a trendy restaurant greets them by name, ushers them to the best table, and whispers in their ear that the fresh oysters are amazing, not on the menu, and they only have a few portions available but will offer them to her/him first, even better.

Budget is not something most average to unhealthy Fours are concerned with, no matter what their financial situation. You can find them obliviously ordering the most expensive meal/wine in the party, without thought for who is paying, simply because that's what they feel like or feel they deserve.

Fours Entertaining at Home

As with their food choices, Fours need their environment to reflect their emotions. The décor, lighting, and music are as important as the food itself. If they feel that their environment can't reflect their love of beauty or whatever they are currently experiencing emotionally, they would rather not entertain.

When asked why he never wanted to have friends over a Four explained: "My house is not the way I would like it to be. There's so much that needs fixing or tidying. As a result, I don't want people to see the clutter and all the broken cupboards and so on. I'd rather not entertain unless my home was the way I'd like it to be, preferably very sparsely furnished but with beautiful exotic pieces."

A Four's home will also reflect their love of beauty, with carefully chosen artworks or décor pieces, maybe even at times verging on minimalistic expression, rather than clutter. They may use their creative energy to create an unusual table decoration and spend ages paging through décor magazines or Pinterest to spark ideas. Incense, candles, exotic music, or fresh flowers may create ambience, invariably with a quirky creative twist. But another time, when their mood is less cheerful, you may find stark decoration and little effort taken. They also like appearing mysterious and exotic, and this can also affect their choice of décor.

The actual presentation of the food is important. It must be beautiful, so they may spend ages perfecting the way the food looks on the plate, adding micro greens or dabs of sauce, if food is where they choose to express their creativity.

But not all Fours are culinary and décor gods/goddesses. If they have a creative outlet elsewhere, a takeout from a trendy restaurant may be as good as it gets. Because the food reflects the mood, if they are down, they may put minimal effort into both décor and preparation. They want you to pick up on this. As hosts, if they have a stronger Type Five wing, they may completely forget to top up guests' wine glasses or offer them coffee, as they are so absorbed in their own conversation or needs.

If you are entertaining a Four, it can be a hard task—what worked for them last month may have evolved into a different diet, so be sure to ask them what they do and don't eat before preparing food, to avoid possible embarrassment.

Food Choices

Fours prefer to shop in delicatessens, *fromageries, patisseries,* Whole Foods and other organic markets, and specialist shops in general, preferably where they are on first-name terms with the owner and/or staff. Shopping is an experience—a time to engage the senses, whether it's a ripe, runny brie or a handmade chocolate. Food choices then become linked to identity and the search for true self. As a result, they may change choices or stores as easily as they would explore different styles of dress.

France is a country where Fours predominate, hence their love of fine food. Think of the exquisite markets in France, where super-fresh produce with beautiful textures and colors are sensuously displayed. French people love to pick up each fruit or vegetable, smell it, feel it, taste a sample, and generally be romanced by its beauty and aroma before purchasing it. They enjoy the juicy interaction with the people selling the food, if they can describe the process by which it's made or list its intriguing ingredients.

Fours are drawn to exotic foods, beautiful packaging, and sensuous colors. For them, it's not a case of buying a simple loaf of bread—Fours look for bread made from stone-ground, organically grown spelt flour slow-leavened with sourdough yeast, artisan crafted in limited quantities and hearth-baked, as a way of experiencing that one exquisite taste. Mass-produced items are not for them, neither are popular brands. Even if they have budget constraints, a Four would rather have coffee only once a day rather than their desired three times a day, if they can enjoy some special brew. They will tell themselves that they are worthy of the best, no matter what the cost, and envy those who can afford a lifestyle where they can always afford these "essential" luxuries.

They may be drawn to retro-type packaging—coffee sold in old tins, biscuits in hessian bags with beautiful ribbons, or ice cream cones that are made from genuine Belgium wafers.

As mentioned, the two types of Fours will act differently. Bohemian[2] Fours may only keep milk and coffee at home and little else, eating out at vegan restaurants or casual eateries while Aristocratic Fours will opt for new upmarket, trendy restaurants and a fridge well stocked with the crafted food they enjoy, in case they entertain, or available simply for their own pleasure. Both types will be drawn to choose food that others will see as different.

For a Four, current experiences are sieved through experiences from the past. Whether it's the music, setting, or a certain dish, they may be drawn into an emotion that occurred in the past when the experience was similar ("Eating crispy duck always reminds me of my last meal with Keith before we ended things. It was very emotional for both of us. We sat in this small restaurant in Taipei, knowing it had to end. Eating the same dish here makes me feel the awful sadness I felt then"). This is a typical Four experience, drawing up the past and blending it with the present. These reminisces can be either happy or sad, but they always elicit a lot of emotion for a Four.

Fours are very aware of the body and its needs and the effect certain foods have on them. They may complain that bread makes them feel bloated and that cheese affects their stomach and sleep patterns. If we believe that our thoughts are intrinsically linked to our physical selves, then it stands to reason that Fours may develop bodies with specific needs that are different to the (lesser) needs of others. As a result, they may complain more of illness and pain—the emotional pain becomes actual physical pain.

The need for specialized foods once again sets them apart from others. In a relationship, this can translate as "my needs are more important than yours," particularly if the Four is married to a less confrontational type, such as a Nine, a Six, or a Two ("We can't eat at the curry place because curries give me heartburn. No, not the pizza place, I'm wheat intolerant. Chinese won't work—the soy sauce gives me an upset stomach"). The other partner is expected to conform to their choice because (it is presumed) they don't suffer equal complaints.

They can annoy others because they have no qualms about cutting off the best part of the meat for themselves or taking the juicy inner part of the pie, whilst leaving the pastry crust for fellow diners. They simply feel entitled to the best bits.

If they choose to be vegetarians, it will be because as sensitive souls, they truly feel for the pain and trauma animals endure to feed us. If their bodies are their temples, then filling them with hormones and antibiotics ingested from meat or chemicals from pre-cooked, ready-made meals would be a concern. Being a vegetarian allows for guilt-free eating.

What You May Not See

Fours may eat little or unconsciously when they become depressed or overabsorbed with feelings of melancholy. It's as if the starvation heightens emotional awareness, which becomes a fix.

"Sometimes I'd go for days without food, because the pain is so strong that hunger has lost its meaning," a Four describes. "I seem unable to deal (correctly) when food's involved. I either binge, restrict, or binge and purge. I can't just ... eat. It doesn't work like that; it's not that easy. Food pretty much controls my life, and that's somewhat intentional as I can't deal with my life, either ... but food—thinking about it, fussing over it, and so on—takes priority over all other aspects of being alive."

Perhaps not as common as with Ones, bulimia and anorexia can become an issue with Fours.

In their desire to be different, and in focusing on what they see as their faults, they may see themselves as exempt from society and its prescribed roles, particularly in earning a living or carrying out responsibilities. They may give up a job to write a book, play, poetry, artwork, or the like, expecting their partner/family member/friend to carry them emotionally and financially while the book is being written (which might just be a very long time, as each word is endlessly honed, researched, and perfected). Any complaints by the partner may result in a hissy fit of note and blame being laid at the other person's door. They have sought and found the "rescuer" who will see to all their needs.

"I wanted to be a musician. By working very hard and supporting the family, my wife allowed me to become one," a Four recalled. What he didn't add, however, was that his wife was not happy with the situation at all and resented having to work 24/7 because she was supporting the family single-handedly. He simply didn't want to see or acknowledge this. He was a musician and so deserved to be left removed from worldly responsibilities to create his art. The music, by his admission was not "mainstream, commercial stuff" so not able to generate an income. Yet at the same time he was angry because his lover was seldom available to him because of her workload.

How They View Their Bodies

Most Fours will be highly critical of what they see as their "flaws." What happens is their imagined emotional flaws get projected onto their bodies. Some Fours see their bodies as their artistic canvas. They can spend hours at the gym, lifting weights and doing exercises to hone each muscle to perfection. Their body is their artwork, to be pampered, worked on, and adorned with tattoos, creams, jewellery—whatever they feel enhances it best.

If they have Three wings, they may, like some Threes be drawn to cosmetic surgery to eliminate their "flaws." When they don't feel much happier after the process, they may focus on another aspect of their physical selves they find unlikeable and require more surgery. As such, surgery can become addictive.

An extreme example of this is the French feminist artist Orlan, who during the 1990's had herself filmed while undergoing cosmetic surgery to alter her appearance in order to look more like Leonardo's Mona Lisa and Botticelli's Venus, among others.

Orlan apparently did not undergo these nine surgical procedures for art's sake us such, but more as an exploration of her need to be different and to reinvent herself as well as to undoubtedly shock society as a result. Unlike other women having cosmetic surgery to correct 'flaws' or to appear younger, exploring news ways of being physically, became her art.

Other Fours may take little interest in their bodies if their creativity becomes their focus, if the canvas is the expression rather than the body.

Addictions

Fours are often intense people and are attracted to drugs that will help calm them down and console them, such as marijuana or cigarettes. They are also often socially insecure, so may drink to make socializing easier, or in the words of Ernest Hemingway, "I drink to make other people more interesting." Antidepressants, sleeping pills, and other prescription drugs, often taken in combination, are not uncommon. They feel they have had a worse deal than anyone else in life and often justify their addictions with this belief. [3]

Addictions bring them relief from feelings of self-hatred. Should they open up in group therapy or drug rehab situations, they will spill their emotional guts, raw and unfettered, onto the group. Having taken an observing backseat, when they do let their emotions loose, they can tend to take over the group and exclude others' participation.

Childhood

Fours frequently report experiencing feeling abandoned[4] as children by both or one of their parents. Most typical is a feeling of being abandoned by their mothers—either because she was experiencing post-partum depression or because she was physically absent (as in death or travel), engrossed with a younger sibling, working, or ill. The feeling of being abandoned then translated into not being worthy of being cared for, misunderstood, unworthy of being loved, and of being defective in some way; hence, the motivation to be noticed—to be seen as not defective, to be special.

If the parent is emotionally absent and ignores the emotional needs of the child, the child may act out to attract the attention they feel they are not receiving. If other siblings seem to be getting the love and attention they crave, being different or dramatic becomes the way they try to make themselves and their feelings heard.

This sense of loss of the beloved parent can translate into the constant search for the beloved other. Perfect love has been lost and translates into a lifelong search for love and the person who "gets" them. They long to be seen as mysterious and elusive, so the beloved (or passing infatuation) will come looking for them, and thereby affirm their significance.

As mentioned, they frequently feel as if they have been born into the wrong family, and the fabulously exotic couple down the road should really have been their parents. This can make them feel isolated, different from their siblings, so they constantly seek an identity for themselves, away from their inherited family environment. If I can't relate or am not like my family/tribe, then who am I?

Because they often feel different from one or both parents or the family, Fours can often have issues with their mothers or maternal figures (which may be male), and this may play out over their whole lifetime. "My mother never loved me like she did my sister and brother. No matter what I did, they always came first," a friend said to me.

They may spend their lives looking for the parent or parents they feel they did not have and often feel let down by those they choose to project these feelings on, leading to bouts of rage. As their neediness and expectations of others increases, they may drive away the very person who was rescuing them, thereby repeating the childhood experience.

Diets for Fours

Popular diets seldom attract Fours, but visiting a dietitian for a personalized diet plan will. Less emotionally healthy Fours are at the mercy of their desires. Add to this the feeling of entitlement, as in "I deserve this," then you can see that dieting can be a tricky issue. As their moods swing, so does their commitment to self-control. They don't see themselves as being beholden to the dietary rules and, as noted earlier, have strong opinions they aren't afraid to share. If you are seeing a Four as a client, you may find that they have strong views on foods, which will most likely not be mainstream.

They often are great nibblers or in-between-meals snackers, forgetting what they have eaten during the day. "I just had a couple of nuts" can mean I ate the packet.

They tend to like doing things at set times ("After yoga, I have a rice cake and hummus—it grounds me—then after lunch, a coffee, which enhances my mood and creates the environment for work and creative activity. At around 5 p.m., I get hungry and have another rice cake and hummus and then a glass of chilled Chardonnay to relax myself. Then it's supper time at 6 p.m."). Here again, it may have actually been four rice cakes and several glasses of wine.

Taking this inclination to nibble into account, any diet aimed at a Four should accommodate the need for healthy snacks between meals.

Fours can be self-indulgent, which conflicts with the regime of a diet. The issue of entitlement arises here: "I need something to stimulate my creativity. Lettuce just won't do it. I long for marzipan dark chocolates made by the chocolaterie in town."

They can also undermine a dietitian's (or exercise coach's) confidence by projecting their perceived failure onto the dietitian who may feel (if they allow themselves to) that they have somehow failed the client, as if the advice given is at fault.[5]

What can get them on track is being inspired to be creative with food, within the limitations of what they can eat. Experimenting with new ways of making hummus or a different twist on a Caesar salad can work well, if they are interested in cooking.

If they are unhealthy emotionally, they can throw all caution to the wind and get into unhealthy routines of binge eating and drinking (or drug taking), partying all night, watching movies, or listening to music and then berating themselves for doing so later.

Exercise

As Fours become less emotionally healthy, their bodies reflect this. Being one of the withdrawn types, they isolate themselves into a fantasy world where they can have the identity they desire. At this level of development, doing group exercise is not going to work for them. They may be totally absorbed with what they see as their physical and emotional defects, yet unwilling to work consistently toward improving them.

They may adopt a persona of "I'm overweight, so get lost! It's who I am. I am different, and I am making a statement about beauty being internal." If they didn't engage in much exercise as children, Fours may be less likely to exercise, particularly if the mood doesn't make them feel inclined to do so on any particular day. Getting into a routine is important, then, if they are to maintain the discipline of exercise. With more than average physical complaints, they may use this as legitimate reason to not show up. Having a fixed routine or clearly defined rules helps keep them on track.

Individualized exercise classes with a spiritual component, such as yoga or Nia dance, may be more popular. Dancing is also a great option as it involves intimacy with others without complications. As one Four described it: "Doing the tango is the most sensual thing you can do. You are exquisitely, intimately connected with a stranger, and for a few minutes, you move as one. After the dance you separate, having had this experience, yet unlike an actual relationship, there is no hurt, no sense of loss."

They are often quite highly strung and so may be drawn to more aesthetic slower exercises, such as surfing, where hours are spent out at sea just contemplating the prospect of the perfect wave. Rowing or canoeing is also an option. They are not particularly competitive and so may enjoy more sports they can do alone, such as rock climbing or hiking.

They may be drawn to a certain exercise routine because of their attraction to the teacher or another class member but then, as quickly as they started, lose the attraction and with it, the class, when they find themselves bored.

How to Inspire Fours

To get Fours on board with any weight-loss or exercise program, they need to see that being more physically fit will improve their chances of finding a partner.[6] Although they are doing it for themselves, if they feel better about themselves and the way they look, that in itself is attractive. Feeling more confident will allow them to connect more intimately with others; they will truly show up, and so will others.

Levels of Health

Healthy

Fours have, as mentioned, an idealized vision of who they would like to be. The healthier they are emotionally, the closer they are to actualizing their fantasy. Their body is their temple and is honored as such. They intuitively know what is best for their bodies. They don't envy others' figures or believe they are more flawed than others, as they do when less healthy. Their sense of self extends way beyond their physical appearance; they attain self-acceptance and have a clear sense of self.

They may explore their feelings but are not self-absorbed; they are kind and sensitive not only to their own but others' feelings. They exude an air of originality, self-awareness, love, and grace. They do what is right for themselves and others and have a presence that is truly transforming. They do not have to do or be anything other than what they already are to experience their own uniqueness.

Average

As Fours become less healthy emotionally, this starts to reflect in their health. The fantasy self and the perceived reality self start drifting farther apart, leaving Fours attempting to create an identity. They look for a rescuer who will see them as they cannot see themselves and start testing those they are in relationship with. The beginnings of self-dislike reflect in poor food choices, and the stirrings of desire for alternative realities where they can feel good can often be enhanced by drugs and alcohol. Trying to get themselves back on track, eating wise, they may be sabotaged by emotional upsets and feelings of "I'm not really worth it."

They may demand endless conversations about the relationship, pointing out where the partner is at fault, while simultaneously becoming needy. They fear being boring, so take actions to create appearance choices that reflect the difference they desire. This can reflect in food choices. Increasingly they feel misunderstood and can become critical and demanding of others while ignoring their own failings.

Unhealthy

As they disintegrate, Fours can develop a wild approach to life. Caution is abandoned, and risk-taking rules in the search of new escapist highs. Alternative lifestyles become attractive and enticing at the expense of their well-being. Like unhealthy Sevens, they'll splash out on French Champagne while leaving the mortgage unpaid, or eat rich foods they know are harmful to their well-being. They start believing they are entitled demi-gods/goddesses, who can act as they want without responsibility or explanation.

They increasingly believe that their lives have been harder than anyone else, which gives them permission to act without responsibility for their actions. The tendency toward self-absorption develops further, and they become preoccupied with a fantasy self that is an idealized version of who they would like to be. As the chasm widens between this idealized self and who they see themselves as actually being, they start to reject anyone who does not support their idealized view of themselves.

As people leave, they may then attempt to win them back through favors, manipulation, or by creating dependencies, in the manner of unhealthy Twos. Doing so increases an unhealthy Four's feelings of isolation and sadness. Life feels wasted and meaningless. They become tired, apathetic, and withdrawn, blaming others for not rescuing them and being dismissive. They may turn increasingly to drugs, alcohol, binge eating, or all three.

Being the most self-aware of the Enneagram types allows Fours a unique opportunity to see when they are disintegrating to less healthy states, and they can use their ability for self-reflection to consciously shift this. Naturally, this is something that all types can do; however, a Four's insight gives them an early-warning-system advantage, allowing them to move into the deep, different, passionate, loving beings they are.

Summary

Type Fours can go from being determined dieters to big bingers in the flash of a mood swing. These extremely sensitive souls can lose weight and maintain it when they start working with their bodies rather than against them, if they can see the beauty of the functioning of every molecule in their bodies and gratefully acknowledge this by acting as guardian of their physical selves and their world.

Life coaching or therapy can help a Four detach their feelings from food and begin to realize that being a drama queen does not indicate deep heart connection but an inability to be emotionally real. Letting go of the fixation that you need to be special in order to have an identity makes living in your own skin much more comfortable and allows you to recognize your actual talents.

Create routines for eating and exercise, and don't allow beliefs about your feelings to arise that lead to self-sabotage. Paradoxically, the more structure you create in your life, the more liberated you'll be to express yourself creatively. Through feeling better about yourself, you will be rewarded with greater intimacy with significant others, because you will feel worthy of this love and appreciation.

Type Five
The Neglectful Nosher or Ruminating Relisher

The Issue

For a Five, neglecting the body in favor of the mind (gaining knowledge) is merely a means to a cerebral end. Food holds little importance and is often eaten sporadically, with little or no concern for nutrition.

Overview of Type Five

Fives are your serious, indifferent, thinking (rather than feeling), curious, independent, innovative types. They love knowledge and spend hours acquiring it, most often in specialist fields. They enjoy observing and researching. Dinner parties, cocktails, and superficial chit-chat bore them. They are happy in their own company, working or investigating their latest project in the sanctity of their study or "man-cave," or at leisure, playing computer games or studying esoteric, often dark or taboo subjects. They don't welcome interruptions or events that take them away from the "project."

Fives have deep insights and inquisitive minds. As such, they are the innovators of the world, connecting dots among various bodies of knowledge in order to find creative solutions. Their minds are clear and uncluttered by emotions. They simply know a lot about a lot of things.

You'll often find them bird-watching[1] or collecting unusual items—old computers, butterflies, or whatever interests them. ("I made a list of the most intelligent people I know and thereby admire," a Five confessed to me.)

Of all the personality types, they are the happiest to be alone and, even in a relationship, the Five will want to have a private study or space where they can be alone and pursue their interests (think of the shed at the bottom of the garden).[2] Whereas the Seven recharges their batteries in company, the Five needs alone time to recharge. They are one of the "fear" numbers (like Type Sixes and Sevens). In Fives, fear shows up as the fear of not knowing enough ("The more I know, the more secure I'll feel"). We have a talk show host here in South Africa who amuses me. Every time someone calls in with a question the host can't answer (and this seldom happens), he makes the caller out to be an idiot and invalidates what is often a perfectly reasonable question.

As they become less healthy, Fives view the landscape of life as a vast arid desert where there is not enough to sustain life and as a result, become fiercely protective of their resources. This particularly applies to their time and space, resenting anything that intrudes on it. This is one of the reasons they tend to avoid going out (this, and the fact that they often feel socially inept).

As they disintegrate, they can become the hermits of the world, living in isolation while working on impractical and outrageous projects. They may often research and fine-tune projects to the point of not completing them or becoming more extreme in their concepts (which none but they can understand). They start viewing others as ignorant idiots. They become argumentative and destructive toward others' viewpoints or beliefs. Eccentric nihilists who resist help and become ever more unstable and eccentric.

Ironically, even as a Five works at moving away from contact and attempts to withdraw from others, particularly when emotional issues arise, in order to heal they actually need to engage with others and connect with their bodies like healthy Eights. A readiness to engage rather than withdraw from others and to share their considerable knowledge in a non-patronizing way is how Fives can move to being the curious, accessible, and highly innovative beings they are.

Career Choices

Fives are often great collectors and researchers and may be professors who specialize in a certain field of expertise or work in information technology as software engineers, database administrators, or creators of computer games. Engineering, astronomy, research science, physics, or statistics are also possible career choices. They are typically found as academics in universities, high school teachers, computer scientists, archaeologists, astronomers, rocket scientists, doctors of nuclear medicine, experts on subjects as obscure as, say, Byzantine art or ancient Greek philosophy—any field where a Five's motto, "Knowledge is power," can be pursued.

Eating Triggers

Fives tend to disassociate from the body and its needs. This translates as being disconnected from emotions and attempting to stuff down any feelings that may have emerged using food. The fear that there is never enough in the world can also trigger eating as a way to hoard food while it's available.

Signs to look for that may indicate stress include a desire to be on their own, neglecting not only their food and food choices but also personal hygiene, and the inability to socially interact with others. They may suffer increasingly from insomnia and entertain increasingly bizarre ideas. Like stressed Fours, they often refuse any assistance and may even become hostile toward those closest to them who want to help them. Suicidal thoughts and depression are common.

How Fives Approach Eating

Fives have the ability to be not aware that they are hungry. They may skip meals because they are so involved in a project or playing a computer game and then, when they are famished, wolf down whatever they can find—chips and a coke, leftovers from a couple of days back, instant pot noodles, cup-a-soup, yesterday's pizza—it really doesn't matter; whatever is available or can be tossed into the microwave. Unless they are chefs themselves, food is of little concern to Fives, which is why they can end up often eating unhealthily. This starve-then-eat habit can lead to binge eating when food is available.

They are quite content to find a certain thing they enjoy and are happy to eat that for every meal. For example, an artist friend of mine, rather than interrupt his work, quite happily lived on cornflakes for each meal because it was cheap and quick and easy to prepare. Food was a task that needed to be done to survive but the rich sensual pleasure available to be explored in creamy red wine sauces and exotic flavor combinations held no interest. Not to say he didn't enjoy a good meal, but rather that he had no attachments to eating. Likewise, another man discovered a certain brand of cottage cheese he enjoyed and would eat that with crackers for lunch every single day.

Fives are the iconoclasts of the personality types, so you can be sure that if the world is advocating no carbohydrates and a high-protein diet, the Five will do research and strongly advocate the opposite; moreover, with the research behind him or her, they will then proceed to discount every diet they come into contact with. As such, they become eccentrics and extremists who may, as they disintegrate, only choose to eat at Burger King every day or eat fish heads with pineapple because they have heard that the combination creates unique health benefits.

I did know a Five who advocated this diet, together with goat's milk and goat's milk yogurt. The goats had to be a special breed, so he bought a couple of goats himself to ensure a regular supply of goat's milk. In the end, he made himself ill. Another example is a friend who is of the belief that fat does not make you fat but does the opposite (this was researched at length). Each lunch and dinner, he sat down happily to a bowl of ice cream and ladles of cream, even after his cholesterol sky-rocketed. Fives can become very argumentative and patronizing toward anyone who disputes their theories.

Fives Eating Out

Next time you're out, notice the guy/girl sitting a bit removed from everyone else and closest to the nearest door/escape hatch. Chances are you will have hit upon the introverted Five in the group.

Fives will be the ones who on hearing they have to go out will be saying: "Do we have to? I feel like going out about as much as I feel like root canal treatment." Often, then, if they are involved in a relationship (and they are the most likely personality type not to be), Fives may barter with their partners by saying things like, "Okay, I'll go, but can we agree to leave by 10 p.m.?" (unless it's a group of their colleagues or an event where they want to be to gain further knowledge, such as meeting a visiting professor, author, and so forth).

Fives mostly prefer to approach you rather than be approached. They'll withdraw from a garrulous guest who overwhelms them. They don't enjoy feeling intruded upon.

If you're into Groupon or other "buy-one-get-one-free" discount vouchers, don't expect a Five to share your enthusiasm. Fives are seldom attracted to coupons, but they may go to a discount warehouse like Costco, where they can stock up and avoid having to waste time shopping again.

Because they are often disinterested or ambivalent about food, going out can seem like a huge waste of money and an annoying waste of time. They may end up ordering the most expensive items on the menu, either because they are completely disinterested in the price or as covert revenge for being made to go out. They don't enjoy sharing their meals, so dipping your fork into their tagliatelle for a taste will likely not be well received.

Fives Entertaining at Home

This could be the shortest section in the book, because most fives are not happy entertaining. They don't feel at ease in company, and while they may tolerate a gathering of close friends, colleagues, or family, a cocktail party with its frivolous superficial talk is enough to have them heading home as soon as is politely possible (or sometimes even when it's not polite).

The exception to this would be the Five who has made a study of cooking and the dinner party is then a place to show off their skills to others. Think of British celebrity chef Heston Marc Blumenthal, OBE and owner of *The Fat Duck*, a three-Michelin-starred restaurant voted Best Restaurant in the UK. He is one of the world's most innovative and revolutionary chefs. One of his books, *Kitchen Chemistry*, rather sums it up. As the title suggests, the book details the chemistry involved in cooking and flavor combining. It's a typically Five-ish way to research, explore, study the nature of food, and emerge with innovations that are eccentric and outlandish.

Blumenthal's signature dishes include Snail Porridge, Bacon and Egg Ice Cream, Mock Turtle soup (which combines a multi-sensory experience with historical references), and Meat Fruit. "He first started looking at historic recipes, particularly recipes from medieval times, and one dish that really attracted his attention, just because it was completely mad. The dish was meat fruit," which was literally meat turned into fruit. People in the Middle Ages believed fruit and vegetables were considered to have diseases unless cooked. With a typically wicked sense of humor, medieval chefs played on this fear by forming and painting meat to make it look like raw fruit. The idea being to shock and delight their diners."

He has pioneered the use of sound as part of the dining experience with his *Sound of the Sea* dish, where diners listen to a recording of the seaside—crashing waves with occasional sounds of distant seagulls, children's laughter, and the horn of a ship—while they eat a dish of king fish, kombu-cured halibut, ballotine of mackerel with five different seaweeds, sea jelly beans, and monk's beard served on "sand" made from tapioca starch, ice cream sugar cone, toasted breadcrumbs, kombu, and baby eels or anchovies.[3]

Because they are preoccupied with the world inside their heads, Fives may appear to be inhospitable—forgetting to refresh drinks glasses or generally seeing to the needs of the other guests. They may get up, make themselves a cup of coffee, but not think to ask if anyone else may also enjoy a cup. It's not because Fives mean to be rude; it simply hasn't occurred to them. They can feel estranged from the world outside of their heads and find it hard to tap into the needs of others.

Their homes may be sparsely furnished with odd collected pieces of furniture. Not being handymen or women, broken things they don't need for work may remain unfixed. What interests them—their collection of old computers or sci-fi film posters—may take pride of place. Practicality is not their strong point!

So you may find yourself eating takeout off the coffee table while sitting on cushions on the floor. Yesterday's dirty dishes (unless they have a partner) may be stacked up in the sink. Yet being able to describe at length the attributes of the various accompanying wines or the exact preparation of a certain exotic foodstuffs, should this be their interest, will have the Five unusually engaged.

A Five's response to there not being enough is to diminish their needs rather than reach out into the world to get more (clients, work, projects, and so forth). Foodwise, this translates into being able to exist on very little, a fact they enjoy because it allows them to feel less attached, more independent.

Desire feels uncomfortable for them; nonattachment is the solution. Shutting themselves off from the desire creates a safe haven. Needs are scary. The fewer their needs, the safer they feel. Not to say they can't enjoy a great meal but the desire for it is what makes them afraid. They may describe this as "treading lightly on the planet," but in truth, it's part of their need to withdraw. They are happiest eating with a partner (just the two of them). If they are not in a relationship, then you'll probably find them eating in front of the computer while doing research or playing a game.

Food Choices

Fives are so self-involved mentally that while they focus on their thesis or attempt to solve a mathematical problem, they will eat anything, oblivious to its taste. They don't mind eating the same foods everyday—indeed, the lack of ambiance around the meal suits them just fine. Their food choices are usually not healthy. An example was my son's college roommate, who ate bread, bacon, and egg for breakfast, lunch, and dinner, with the odd pizza thrown in. When the roommate's health deteriorated as a result, his parents were forced to organize meal delivery to the dorm.

The exception to this lack of interest in food is if they get interested in a certain type of food and become expert in it. Take cheese, for instance. A Five may research various cheeses, their origins, how they are made, and so on, and take pride in serving a variety of cheeses to guests and discussing their various attributes. They'll enjoy visiting the dairy farms where the various cheeses are made and talking with the cheesemakers to pick up more valuable information. They may read up on the history of cheese-making, in order to further understand the process.

Should Fives become vegetarian, it will most likely be because they have researched the negative long-term effects of being carnivores, such as a greater chance of getting Type 2 diabetes, Alzheimer's disease, and so forth. Practically speaking, it can also be because it's generally cheaper to eat vegetarian food—a cup of rice and lentils goes a long way to filling you.

Their particular wound is avarice, or greed. One of the ways this can play out is feeling the need to stock up on piles of non-perishable food so they don't have to worry about shopping any time soon. Shopping is an inconvenience that wastes time they could have spent on whatever project is inspiring them currently.

Fives minimize their physical needs, and this includes food. Doing so takes the stress out of having to choose what to eat. They may skip meals, eat at random times, and snack on a strange variety of easily accessible foods. Snacking is going to win hands down over a full meal, simply because it's usually faster and easier to prepare a snack. Grabbing a packet of chips and crunching on them is easy to do while working.

They may become food hoarders, convinced that some doomsday prophecy will require a store room of canned foods. Or the increasing cost of food may have them hoarding as a means of saving. Fear translates into the Passion of Avarice—there is not enough, so they need to hold onto what they have. Not grasping or holding onto things could result in disastrous poverty or even starvation.[4]

What You May Not See

Fives are in a dilemma. They don't want others to impact on their space and time, yet they long (mostly unconsciously) for human connection. It's a push-pull issue that, like tortoises, has them creeping out of their shells to connect, only to withdraw quickly if they sense they are becoming needy or too dependent on anyone else or someone is becoming too dependent on them.

They absolutely hate not having all the answers, so going to see a dietitian with the idea that they don't already have all the answers to achieve successful weight loss will be extremely difficult. ("I hated not knowing the answers to my kid's random questions about life, the universe, and everything in between. Even if I didn't have the answer to why flies were created, I'd create my own (untruthful) answer rather than say I didn't know.") They are sometimes not quite as intelligent as they would have you believe.

They often have dark interests in religion or their studies. "I wanted to know what drives people to kill," said one university lecturer. "I studied all the books on murder, trying to fathom it out." They are also known as iconoclasts because of their need to debunk popular theories or beliefs.

As they disintegrate, they compartmentalize their lives so that one person may be completely unaware of an aspect known to another about the Five. Sometimes, these different aspects are only revealed at death.

How They View Their Bodies

Fives generally do not have a healthy sense of their bodies and can feel quite nihilistic toward their physical selves. Bodies are simply there to support the brain function. They may have been the nerd at school who never made it into the sporting teams and from then on, they have disregarded their bodies. Unhealthy Fives become like talking heads.

Their outward appearance is of little importance to them, so personal grooming may be an issue.[5] They abhor fashion trends and may be comfortable wearing the same outfits repeatedly. Clothes are not an issue. They may have strange ideas, such as "washing your hair makes it greasier, so if you stop washing your hair, over time it will sort its grease problem out and then you'll never need to wash it again" was one of the theories a Five confided in me. Another Five would head to the beach showers when he wanted to shower, even though the water was always cold. He said it saved him paying for water in his home. The body is not viewed as something that will help them achieve anything in the world. It's viewed as being unimportant. This is most noticeable in female Fives, who may sport practical haircuts and clothing, rather than make any attempt to appear alluring—it's typical iconoclastic Five behavior to move away from social norms.

Addictions

Caffeine and nicotine are popular addictions as they provide a quick stimulus to allow the Five to work, research, or play computer games for longer. They often suffer from insomnia, so feeling sleepy after a bad night can be rectified with a rush of a caffeinated soda or coffee. Sugar is also a common choice, as in chocolates or snack bars or they may get addicted to sleeping pills.

They may also enjoy both "uppers" and "downers" in terms of drug usage. For the "uppers," it could either be a legal prescription, such as Ritalin, or something like cocaine. Fives are often very tense and hyperactive, so they use narcotics such as marijuana to relax and calm them or prescription drugs such as Xanax or Prozac.

In rehab, iconoclastic Fives may challenge recovery methods or try to destroy or challenge the principles they are being taught. In this role, they can be both argumentative and aggressive. They may find other people in rehab mindless and be patronizing about their attempts to follow the course—to the point of rejecting everyone else and being the loner, a position they are comfortable in. It's as if they want others not to succeed. When Fives are this unhealthy, they can be cruel and biting in their honesty, for example, if they have an interest in the darker or even shocking aspects of life, they may expound on the value of taking drugs, making every non-partaker appear foolish.

Childhood

At some point in childhood, Fives decided that to become independent from their maternal figure they had to be able to get to a point of not needing to be nurtured by her. So they adopted a stance of not allowing themselves to want emotional or nurturing interaction from their mothers, focusing instead on developing their intellect.[6] They start learning to hide their feelings under a thick layer of intellect, knowledge and indifference. Mind supersedes heart. The maternal figure may have felt overpowering or intrusive, not understanding the child's boundaries, so they felt the need to isolate in order to protect themselves. They learnt to avoid what they really were longing for. The same applies to food.

Typically, they may be advanced in some areas of learning, yet display a lack of emotional maturity in their peer group. Playing music, collecting bugs, reading—they will gravitate toward any activity where they can focus on their need for space and avoid intrusion.

Diets for Fives

Fives do not want to be dependent on anything or anyone. Food being a form of dependence then creates the dilemma of *I need to eat, but I don't want to be dependent or desirous of any food.*

Fives want to be self-sufficient. Books like *Five Acres and Independence* by MG Kairns or the *The Concise Guide to Self-Sufficiency* by John Seymour have surely been written by Fives for Fives. "The more food (nurturing) becomes inconsequential in my life, the less I fear not having it," said one Five.

Scarcity is a major factor in the Five's belief system. Being in many ways the symbol of scarcity, a diet is therefore going to push uncomfortable buttons. Abundant eating of what is good for you, however, has a far better chance of working. Remember that the reason Fives put on weight is often because they are eating the wrong foods rather than excess food.

The most easily prepared option will work for most Fives; weighing food and recording measurements of their bodies won't. Remember: a Five's fixation is the result of stinginess (the Passion is avarice), so it's doubtful that they will fork out loads of cash on health food options because eating healthily most often is perceived as costing considerably more.

If a Five gets sufficiently interested in researching diets or foodstuffs, in their endearingly eccentric way, they may combine this with an eating plan. For instance, if a Five has done research on the harmful effects of wheat on the body's metabolism, they will be able to expound at great length about the way wheat has changed over the years and the effect wheat has on one's gluten levels. Turning a diet into a study or opportunity for research may intrigue a Five enough to take it up as their latest project, thereby satisfying the dietitian's need to improve the way a Five eats and the Five at the same time.

As is common with Fives, though, expect the quirky. The rare goats' cheese made from certain goats and prepared in a certain way that has unique health benefits. Hemp milk, which has loads of healthy omega-3 fatty acids, iron, calcium and other minerals, vitamins, and acids, may become the flavor of the month, and the Five will happily drink it morning, noon, and night. I knew a Five who spent close to $250 on a single purchase of fresh cherries, because he'd read about their benefits for arthritis.

We should reiterate: Fives hate not knowing things. Should they adopt an eating program, they'll have studied up on every aspect of it so that they don't appear incompetent and unknowledgeable. They will typically go for outlandish ideas and complex theories regarding diets and defend their stance while arguing that every other diet is a waste of time. As noted earlier, overeating can be a mindless action but is a subconscious attempt to feed their inner emptiness and loneliness.

Exercise

Exercising the mind is infinitely more important than exercising the body for a Five. They find greater solace and trust in the power of the mind than that of the power of the body. [7] If their attention is focused on solving a problem, constructing a theory, or playing *World of Warcraft*, they may completely forget their gym appointment or commitment to cycle (and it won't worry them too much).

Fives are not team sports people, so if they do have a sport they enjoy, it will likely be a solitary one. If ornithology, entomology, or outdoor photography counted as sports, I suspect they would be the most popular Five outdoor activities. Fives prefer observing to participating. They may be able to list every victory of the team they support, the score, small details of the match, and so on, and be competitive in demonstrating that knowledge, but they themselves do not play.

"I dreaded after-school sport. It was compulsory, and there were limits to the illnesses I could create just before the last period lesson before sport practice would begin. From a young age, I was inept and weak at sport, so the other kids would tease me. To this day, I have a dread of gyms. But I took revenge in the classroom, where my academic prowess had those same kids floundering," one Five reflected.

A Five's lack of athletic prowess means they often head into unusual sports. Take the unicycle rider I often see balancing precariously on the top of his contraption. I suspect that if I engaged with him, he'd be able to tell me all about the history of the unicycle and possibly infer that as unicyclists go (all four of them in the city!) he was right up there!

They avoid taking action and being strong, in case taking a stand makes them appear foolish. So were they to be in a team, they would not enjoy being the captain, where the need to act and be decisive are imperative. They need time to ponder before deciding on a course of action, so it's chess rather than rugby or football for many of them. They do sometimes become active in sports such as cycling, surfing, hiking, or long-distance running, where they can compete against themselves and have the time to ponder and retreat from the world.

Their bodies often reflect this withdrawal from the physical, by being round-shouldered, spindly, or frail-ectomorphic. They can neglect their bodies and look down on those who make fitness a priority.

Solving some complex problem will be just the excuse they need to avoid exercise.

How to Inspire Fives

If you're a dietitian working with a Five, you're in for an interesting time! Fives will typically question all you propose and have probably researched weight loss in depth, much of which may be controversial. (They may even have found some snippets of off-beat research you've not heard about!) They may argue and attempt to belittle your information and approach, questioning why, in the greater scheme of things, weight loss is even an issue. "What's the point, when we're all going to die of something anyhow" may be their take, unless you have their buy-in.

From a dietitian's point of view, getting a Five interested in the thinking or technical information behind certain food products is the way to inspire them to eat differently. Knowledge to a Five is power, so give them knowledge and encourage them to research further and you'll have an eating convert. But be warned, they may zone out as a means of avoiding what they don't want to accept or acknowledge.

Fives want to be competent and capable. [8] But living life in an unbalanced way, that is, focusing only on whatever project they are busy on, is not leading a balanced life. Withdrawing from others is an indication of incompetency in the world. If you can bring awareness to the issue that says being competent involves a multifaceted lifestyle, being more capable of doing more things, you may be able to inspire them to get on board with the program.

They've likely come from a place of feeling incapable when it comes to sport, but what if they found something they could do. Hike and watch birds? Surf and study wave patterns? Run and give themselves the space to solve the algorithm? As people, they would be more competent and capable. If they improved their eating habits, they would have more energy to see projects through, more confidence to attract a partner, and without health issues, more time to focus on the project.

Levels of Health

Healthy

Fully functioning Fives are focused, innovative, kind, profound, and perceptive. They have a wry or whimsical, understated sense of humor. They are the visionaries and pioneering thinkers of the world, observing it with curiosity but feeling part of it. Being fully grounded and connected with their bodies, they eat consciously and with awareness. While probably not set on being top athletes, they may enjoy outdoor activities such as hiking or bird-watching, which give them time to study and reflect on new ideas and "join the dots" among different bodies of thoughts. They share their knowledge openly with the world. They "get" ideas and concepts. They love finding out about things and are both curious and clear-minded. If a dietitian explains the functioning of the body and its current limitations, they'll grasp what to do to reverse the process.

Average

Average healthy Fives have started to lose connection to their physical selves. The body is a necessity, a functioning robot-type creature. Fear being an issue, they begin to doubt that they know enough and so throw themselves into gaining knowledge while simultaneously becoming out of touch with their physical needs. Being highly strung, unconscious eating and poor eating habits develop, but potential weight gain as a result can be burnt off by sheer nervous energy (they sometimes have the habit of a leg that twitches rapidly). Food has become a necessary fuel for their functioning, and little more.

Exercise routines may be disregarded in the constant need for research and time allocated to whatever project they are currently working on. Lack of sleep leads to increased nervousness, and they can become antagonistic and derogatory to others who don't share their views or who don't understand them. "Exercise is for idiots who don't have anything more important to do!" "It's been proved that dieting puts more stress on the body than poor eating habits" are the kinds of obscure arguments they put forward.

Unhealthy

As Fives move into less healthy emotional states, they become more identified with their heads and often lose connection to their bodies, to the point that they may forget to take regular meals, exercise, or even to follow a basic hygiene routine. How this translates into their eating patterns is that they may skip meals or eat while working. A typical scenario would be the computer geek playing games through the night and ordering-in takeout pizza, which he can eat while continuing to play. These unhealthy eating habits may lead to weight gain, or alternatively, if the Five is so focused on work, gaming, and the like that they skip meals, they may become thin, wisplike, and malnourished.

I worked with one Five who, after entering a state of relaxation, described to me how he had an imaginary wall around himself, much like a medieval castle wall (as a way of keeping others out of his inner world). When we discussed the effect this had on his life, he agreed to go away and spend time visualizing breaking down parts of the "wall." Several weeks later, I inquired about how this was working for him, and he replied that he first had to source a mental "tractor" to help with the process, and this was taking some time!

As Fives disintegrate, nihilism can enter the picture, and they may neglect the body and feel that any kind of healthy bodily practice is pointless, just as they feel all existence is.

Disintegration is usually unconscious but to become healthier often requires conscious effort. Fives need to let go of their avarice cage—where they feel that there is never enough so that what they have needs to be stored, from ideas, cash, and cardboard to resources and time—and experience the abundance in the universe. Knowledge cannot buy the power of true gnosis. Life mastery is seldom obtained through books. When Fives stop trying to outsmart others and awaken to their own inner depth and observant minds, they can access profound insights and join the dots among different concepts, to create innovative solutions to the world's problems (and their own).

Summary

Fives need to learn to reconnect with their physical and emotional selves. They need to understand that using their minds can be a defense against feeling their emotions and being in their physical bodies; that true knowledge is the knowledge of oneself and one's emotions; that is, an inner knowing rather than purely knowledge of things external. They must learn to believe in the bounty of the world, starting with nature, and understand that their need to isolate themselves is born of fear not of having no need of others. That reaching out, although hard, offers true nonattachment; that there can be no true learning that does not involve the heart, and knowledge is worthless unless it's shared.

Type Six

The Fight-or-Flight Feaster or Courageous Culinarian

The Issue

Sixes have fear as their major wounding; put another way, fear is what stops them from being present, because fear projects us into the future—what may happen. Faced with a terror, fight or flight becomes a Six's way of coping, resulting in them subconsciously either keeping trim and fit so they can run in the face of danger (flight) or gaining weight so nobody will mess with them (fight). Anxiety triggers overindulgence, be it with food, drugs, or alcohol.

Overview of Type Six

The Yiddish word *mensch* is a great word to describe a Six. They are the backbone of society—hard-working, loyal, responsible, engaging, dutiful, and good at organizing. They are the glue that holds a family, army, organization, or corporation together. They enjoy a stable, safe environment and are usually good team workers (provided that the rest of the team is pulling alongside them). They don't do well when they feel others are slacking. They can have a great self-deprecating humor, which is why you'll often find comedians who are Sixes. They do this so that they appear as no threat to others—they want to say, "Hey, it's safe with me."

Sixes are often the most difficult of the types to identify, because they come in such a wide variety of forms and can be ambiguous, presenting as one thing one day and another, the next. Because of this duality, Sixes can "walk in another's shoes" and truly see issues from another person's perspective. This makes them generally compassionate people, because they "get" where the other person is coming from. It can also make them take up the opposing cause, hence the term devil's advocate is often associated with them.

It is commonly acknowledged that Sixes are constantly scanning the horizon for what could potentially go wrong. It's as if by thinking of all the worst-case scenarios, a Six attempts to prevent them from occurring. They're the type who actually reads the airplane guide as to what to do in the case of an emergency and know where all the exits are.[1]

They are afraid of certain authority figures, which may differ from one Six to another. This results in them exhibiting the opposite behavior; for example, acting the rebel to prove to themselves that they aren't afraid.

Courage is an issue with Sixes. As they integrate, they find the courage to work through their fears, and at healthy levels, they can sometimes even look like the classic hero/ine. They have a deep sense of intuitive knowing, are well grounded with inspirational inner strength. Once they make you their friend, they are committed and loyal in the extreme.

Counter-phobia (going against the natural wounding of each type) exists in all Enneagram types but is most obvious in certain Sixes who, in an attempt not to appear afraid, go toward the fear rather than run from it. So, it's the guy or girl who kayaks through remote areas alone, bungee jumps or rides massive waves, all the while being afraid. While many Sixes adhere to safety and security, the counter-phobic Six does just the opposite. Take, for example, South African professional soccer player Ryan Botha who, on seeing a man fall 8 meters into a swimming pool, leapt two stories to the ground, breaking both a leg and an ankle, to help save the man. Courage is won through action despite fear.

At average health levels, Sixes start looking for reassurance from others about their decisions. They may take on more work (to feel safer in their job), yet complain about it. They start to test the loyalty of others and find their heads can become a cacophony of conflicting inner voices telling them what action to take.[2]

When unhealthy, Sixes become more reactive and can adopt "divide and rule" behavior, as they become suspicious of all around them and don't know who can be trusted. Because trust is something Sixes find hard, both of themselves (they usually suffer from low self-esteem) and of others, they often see things that aren't real, projecting their neurosis onto others. *There must be a motive at work here. They can't simply be doing what they are doing to be nice* would be a typical thought of a less healthy Six. As a result, they often test relationships by provoking a potential friend, just to see if they will return—if they can be relied upon.

When unhealthy, Sixes can become defensive, paranoiac, and increasingly anxious. They can push others away only to feel even more insecure afterwards. Their behavior becomes increasingly hard to fathom and in their panic, they may imagine enemies everywhere. Conspiracy theories abound. The world becomes a dangerous place where no-one can be trusted.

But life doesn't have to unfold like this. Sixes can move toward their healthy engaged selves, where they truly learn to have trust, both in themselves and others. They can act in spite of their fear, knowing that they have the support of the universe. As such, they are trusting, often funny, and intuitive.

Career Choices

Their ability to relate to others' insecurities makes Sixes excellent therapists, alternative healers, and counselors. They are thinking types, however, and tend to intellectualize their feelings rather than actually feel them. They want to be of service to the world and to help others. They like to be seen as someone you can rely on, so you'll find them as bankers, health care workers, social workers, teachers, police officers, in the army, philosophers, security guards, police detectives—anywhere they can support others and feel supported themselves. They are often creative. They enjoy solving problems, so you'll also find them as troubleshooters, statisticians, solving IT-related problems, and in jobs managing risk (although not at their own personal risk). They are cautious, reliable, and enjoy detail. This ability to check out potential problems makes Sixes great scenario planners.

How Sixes Approach Eating

Like Ones, Sixes eat with a conscience but for a different reason. Ones may not eat meat because it's the right and moral thing to do, whereas Sixes will do so out of genuine empathy for the animal. "Eating meat is unhealthy and adds to your cholesterol level," (Type One) versus "I don't eat anything with a face; I can't bear the thought of how the animals suffer," (Type Six).

They may be very suspicious of foods they have not tasted before, particularly exotic foods or foods from a different culture. If meat and three vegetables was what they experienced in childhood, then that's what they'll feel most comfortable with in adulthood. Food reminiscent of the past can make them feel secure—safe, comfort food.

They can also be very definite about what they do and don't like ("I never ate peas as a child, and I still don't"). This rigidity in food choices can be unhealthy, dependent on what foods they reject. "I won't eat 'rabbit' food" (greens) may mean that they end up being deficient in vital vitamins and minerals.

Meal times tend to be regular, so they'll eat at a certain time, even if they aren't particularly hungry. Sixes can also overeat as a type of insurance policy—eat now because you never know when there won't be food available. It sounds ludicrous, and Sixes would agree, but deep in their subconscious this fear of lack lurks.

One Six said: "I always finish my plate, even if I am full, because that's the way I was brought up. But when I thought about it, my siblings don't do that, so I realized it had more to do with me than my upbringing. It's as if I'm afraid that there may not be another meal, as if I'm eating as if this was my last supper."

When fear starts arising, when they are stressed and overworked, when they doubt themselves, or are looking for ways to procrastinate, eating can become a way of alleviating that stress. Even if it's at a social function where they feel unsure of themselves, tucking into the snacks helps to calm them but has a detrimental effect on their health and waistline.

Sixes, as mentioned, are both the rebels as well as conformists of the Enneagram. So you can have the ambiguity arising, where one rebel "voice" is telling them to eat more and another conformist voice telling them to restrict themselves.

Eating Triggers

What indicates that a Type Six may be suffering from serious stress that will trigger poor eating habits? Knowing what we do regarding a Six's relationship to fear, panic attacks and intense anxiety are indications that they are experiencing high stress levels,[3] which the anxiety will further increase in a vicious circle. To this add depression and low self-esteem, ambiguously combined with verbally attacking those closest to them, fearing all the while that they will lose those people's support.

If you're a Six and your wounding involves a fear of what might happen, as your stress levels increase, fear may take the form of thinking that you might not have enough to eat in the days ahead. As noted above, this can lead to overeating today in a squirrel-type eating pattern. It's not the "waste not, want not" of Type One but rather a hoarding-type thinking: *If I eat lots today, then I'll have enough to carry me through the following days, if food is scarcer.* This is truer of a Type Six with a Five wing.

Low self-esteem also can lead to binge eating as a form of comfort (*None of these diets work, and no one appreciates me, no matter what I do, so I may as well make myself happier*—through alcohol, food, and so forth).

Sixes Eating Out

Sixes love sharing information on the latest restaurants or the new whisky bar, particularly those Sixes who lean toward a Seven. They tend, though, to be more safe in their food choices, so would be more likely to choose a restaurant serving more traditional dishes than trying a new fad. The "phone a friend" part of a popular quiz program applies very much to Sixes. Because they often don't trust their own judgment, they enjoy getting confirmation from another party as to their menu or restaurant choice ("What do you think of the Beef Wellington? Have you had it here before? Should we go to Carluccio's or Domingo's?"). They want to make a decision but get annoyed with a partner who also doesn't want to risk a decision that may turn out not to have been a good one. This is one of the reasons I suspect that Six women are attracted to decisive Eight men.

They will often order the same meal every time they go to a particular restaurant, rather than risk disappointment with trying something new.[4] However, as with experimenting, the more they lean toward their Sevenish side, the more open they'll be to new choices.

You'll find that most Sixes prefer large picnics or barbeques in the countryside, watching sports matches with mates, and eating at old-style diners rather than fine dining. Sixes love being part of a group or team, so may feel much happier surrounded by friends, colleagues, or family at a restaurant, rather than just being a couple. But once again, as much as I attempt to define Sixes, as I write, I can already think of a couple of Sixes who would prefer an intimate diner for two. With Sixes, the exception rules!

Sixes Entertaining at Home

As a rule, Sixes are family oriented, so it's likely that much of their entertaining will center around their loved ones, with guests as an addition. They may also enjoy inviting team mates round to watch the game or having close friends for a barbeque. They are warm and hospitable, and normally organized when it comes to entertaining.

Typically, they find cooking relaxing and a way to mingle safely with others. They are normally very competent in the kitchen and love nurturing others with what they prepare.

Their kitchens will be functional, with possibly hints of their history—the eggbeater that belonged to granny, the rolling pin that was Mum's, and so on. They like to potter and can spend way too long tinkering with this and that in the kitchen. They are more likely (and this will also depend on their partner) to have a sensible and traditional approach to décor. Images of family, relations, or even photos showing them as part of a team may adorn the living space. They are generally informal in their approach to entertaining, and you may find yourself sitting at the large wooden kitchen table, rather than in a delicately decorated dining room.

Food Choices

Sixes tend to prefer hearty, home-cooked food. They enjoy eating, so what they make will have a sensual quality to it, such as rich soups, casseroles, and so forth. They tend to follow recipes closely, often lacking the confidence required to experiment. They are creative, though, so although they take a traditional approach, you may find interesting additions, such as a gremolata sprinkled on the beef stew or pesto on a vegetable.

They often speak of hearing chatter inside their heads—usually voices from relations or authority figures.[5] These "voices" tell them what they should and should not be doing. The meditation term "monkey mind" describes it well. When the directions from these voices are in conflict, it can become very confusing for a Six to decide what to eat. There are so many opinions. Which should they choose or listen to? Hence the need to call on another person for input.

Sixes are excellent at optimizing, so they'll find out where the best deal is or what coupon to use. They gravitate toward tried-and-tested brands, often selecting products they had as a child, making them the most brand-loyal of the Enneagram types.

What You May Not See

Sixes can be prone to overeating when in a social situation, either because they are anxious and food helps relieve the anxiety or because that was the portion size they grew up on. They can, in their orderly, responsible way, appear to be Ones, but their desire for order is not because it's the right thing to do but more about trying to make their world an ordered and thus safer place to live in. They may have thought of what could go wrong when they were entertaining and now work hard to alleviate these possible disasters.

But life, as we know, often dishes up our issues. A good example is a dear Six friend who offered to host a class reunion. With people who have not seen each other in 30 years, there's bound to be some awkwardness, but things seemed to be going relatively smoothly. Phew! They were having a barbeque, and everyone had brought their own meat. The fire was lit and the salads made. Everything was under control. That is until her guard dog (Sixes love guard dogs) [6] made her way into the kitchen and scoffed all the meat—every sausage and piece of steak! Her worst fears had manifest, just not in a way she could possibly have foreseen.

Sixes have a need to consult authority figures and in a food context, this can relate to finding a particular chef whose recipes they follow religiously. It can also translate as the need to consult with someone regarding the proposed menu (or more often several people).

Sixes can create situations in their minds that aren't true, such as imagining they have done something wrong or that someone dislikes them or their food. They try to second-guess themselves and others and can project what they feel or fear onto others (*Susan hated the curry, I'm sure*). Often those around them are completely unaware of this inner turmoil.

How They View Their Bodies

Sixes traditionally suffer from low self-esteem. This plays out strongly in relation to how they feel about their bodies. No matter how often they go to the gym or exercise, no matter how trim they are, they'll still have a sense of not being good enough. They may believe that their bodies are not to be trusted, as if somehow their body will or has failed them; that they constantly need to test their bodies to ensure that they won't be let down by them.

Being fear types, Sixes will often try to counteract these fears by carrying weapons. Other Sixes may protect themselves with mace spray, stun guns, or by bodybuilding to look imposing. Another means would be to join a gang, the army, police force, a religious group, or any other organization where safety happens in numbers.

With self-esteem issues and feeling uncertain of themselves, and not comfortable in their own skin, they may seek to compare their bodies with colleagues, family, and friends. (*Am I the fat one in the group? Do I have more cellulite than Joan? Are my mates' biceps all larger than my own?*)

Six women often date/marry Type Eight men, who they feel will protect them, even if it does mean sacrificing some of their freedom to the dominating Eight.

Because they are group people and can feel their own opinion has little value, they tend to go along with the group's view on bodies. If they are part of a culture of say IT nerds whose preoccupation is computer game playing, then they will probably adopt the group's lack of body interest. If, on the other hand, they are part of a beautiful people jet-set group, then their bodies will become a full-time occupation and preoccupation, resulting in cosmetic surgery and the like.

Variations in Body Types in Sixes

Enneagram types can be split into further subsections. As mentioned in the first section of the book, one subsection breaks down types into the instinctual priorities of Self-Preservation, Social, or Sexual. These three splits and the flavor each one gives to the different Enneagram types is the work of an entire book, but they have relevance with regard to the body-type for Sixes, hence my need to touch on them here.

The Self-Preservation Type Six is the much warmer of the three categories of Sixes.[7] More like Nines, they believe that overcoming fear is found in being friendly with others. They often then have more cuddly physiques, which can sometimes mean that they are confused with Nines or Twos.

The Social Six seeks safety in groups or organizations, often admiring the leader of these groups. They also find safety in ideas and philosophies.[8] They know the rules and may shun those who aren't in the group; as such, they can be confused with Type Ones. Here is a quote from a Social Six regarding weight loss: "I was shocked to find that my bodyfat percentage was nearly 25 percent. I immediately researched (Five wing!) how to improve this. Once I found a system of eating and exercising that seemed trustworthy, I latched onto it. In both cases, it wasn't just that I had rules to follow; it was that the rules actually brought me in touch with a sense of purpose and comfort." Because they can tend to overemphasize the importance of the team or social structure, they excel in team sports. They tend to be slim and long-boned—leaner rather than muscular, like Sexual Sixes.

The Sexual type (and here it must be noted that the word "sexual" indicates more of a desire for individual contact) is the counter-phobic Six type, meaning they externalize their fears, acting in such a way as to prove to themselves that they are not afraid. They move against the Six's basic fixation with fear in order to appear strong and create fear in others, rather than feel fear themselves (fight or flight).[9] Because of this, they often appear similar to confrontational Eights. Sexual Sixes are typically physically strong and athletic, and you'll find many of them at the gym, lifting weights, and working out. A good example of this type of Six is Sylvester Stallone (who is believed to be a Six with a Seven wing).

Addictions

Sixes can be workaholics, fearing that unless they are responsible and get the job done, they may lose the job. To keep themselves going, coffee and even amphetamines may become addictions. All this coffee and "uppers" makes them more anxious, though, so to deaden the fear, as well as their busy mind, they may be drawn to "downers" and alcohol. So once again, you get the ambiguity.

Sixes are particularly drawn to alcohol.[10] It soothes frayed nerves and anxiety, although, paradoxically, being drunk can create greater fears for a Six, so the circle perpetuates itself.

Sixes, like Fours and Fives, are prone to depression. They use anti-depressants to attempt to stave off panic attacks and general feelings of lack of self-worth and anxiety.

Sixes may be regulars at the local pub or sports bar, known and liked by friends and patrons as well as social types at community events. Consequently, it can be hard to abstain from drinking because much of their social life revolves around it. In the time it takes to down the first drink, they start to feel more relaxed, part of the vibe, and have a sense of belonging, which translates as security.

If they attend recovery addiction programs, they will be both supportive and compassionate toward others in the program. They may appear to take the teachings onboard, but remember: there's a rebel and saboteur in the Six, edging them toward slipping back into bad habits. This is particularly true if the organization is one that oozes authority. *I'll show you*, goads the insistent voice inside their head, only to have their fear of authority pushing them back on the path. To recover, they will need to understand this link between religiousness, anxiety and the desire to use drink or drugs to deaden it.

Bulimia is more commonly found in Sixes, as well as Type Ones.

"Food," a Six told me, "means stability, safety, and grounding for me because it symbolizes family, home, love, being held, and nourished. Because my mum left me when I was two. I experience my bulimia as giving in and then taking charge and control of my weakness. It's a push/pull experience. Food grounds me and makes me feel safe, but then I feel worthless, lethargic, and disconnected, so the food needs to come out to make space to reconnect inwards. Vomiting is letting go and hoping in doing so to find space and inner guidance in the empty space. Vomiting is exhausting, yet it calms my anxiety. I become clearer, more focused, and able to see inner truths as a result. Interestingly, although my sister, who is a year younger than myself, and I were separated when she was one year old and I was two, we both started binge eating and vomiting at 15 and 16, respectively."

Childhood

So where did this fear come from? Why do Sixes feel that they need to suppress this constant rising fear with food and alcohol? At around the age of two, we start becoming aware that our prime nurturing figure (usually our mother) is separate from us, that we are not one with her. This can be scary, as we experience the world as a separate being.

As we know, the most primal fear in humans and many animals is that of being abandoned. Our prime paternal figure (usually the father, but not always) steps in at this stage to provide the external support. "Jump," says the father. "I'll catch you. I'll protect you."

But what if there was no paternal figure? Or the paternal figure was physically or emotionally absent? Who would catch us? Who would make the world safe? Who would be there to guide us? That's where Sixes stumble, which results in them experiencing the world as a place not to be trusted. People become untrustworthy, and perhaps the greatest issue is that we feel we cannot trust ourselves. In summary, then, the Six experienced the lack (physically or emotionally) of a paternal figure at a crucial age and as a result they learnt not to trust.

It's also common for Sixes to describe childhoods that were emotionally unstable, with one or both parents experienced as unpredictable, either as a result of alcohol, mood swings, or quick to anger.[11]

Diets for Sixes

If you are a dietitian or doctor treating a Six, it's good to be aware of this duality, they feel toward authoritarian figures, which a Six could potentially see you as being. One part of them will want to rebel against your advice, while another part may be terrified that you'll catch them cheating on the diet.

"I know I avoided all my dietitian's and doctor's advice," said a Six. "It was as if I deliberately wanted to sabotage myself, by doing the very opposite of what had been told to me. It was particularly relevant when it came to so-called 'bad' foods and alcohol. When I ended up sitting next to my doctor at a wedding, I didn't want to even sip the Champagne or eat the dessert. I didn't want to anger him, when in all probability, he would not have even noticed."

Sixes may appear compliant, but if not healthy, this compliance masks a rebel who is about to emerge.

In the sea of diets and diet-related books, Sixes can be drawn to certain religions or groups that appear to offer the solution. They are looking for the authority they feel the group represents. Most often, they end up feeling badly let down when what was promised seldom materializes, or the guru is found to live in contrast to what he or she preaches.[12]

While Sixes will enjoy being part of a weight-loss program, with group weigh-ins and so forth, they may become quickly mistrusting if results don't happen fast. Because they are more often traditional in their eating habits, they can resist being made to change eating patterns and may look for a diet where they don't have to change the way they are doing things.

To get them to trust the program, Sixes need to meet people for whom it has worked, people they can trust. Like Doubting Thomases, they need evidence that the program works. It's also essential for them to understand the anxiety that triggers their overeating.

One Six told me: "I tried eating before I went to a cocktail party. I must go to a lot of functions as part of my job. So I'd arrive full, but within minutes I was 'unconsciously' grabbing at whatever snacks were being served. I didn't even want to begin to count how much I'd eaten and drunk at the end of an evening. I never related my stuffing food down with it being an attempt to calm me and quell my anxiety. I thought everyone else was as anxious as I was."

If the Six has gained weight to subconsciously look imposing (so they can "throw their weight around"—attack as a form of defence), then this issue of fear will have to be dealt with first, otherwise you'll have one side of them wanting to lose weight and a stronger neural pathway telling them that they need to look big and imposing to feel safe.

As far as instinctual types go: Self-Preservation Sixes would focus on essential needs and perceived threats; Social Sixes on creating community and social structures; and Sexual Sixes on one-to-one relationships. This will obviously impact on which sub-type is more prone to weight gain and obviously, from an exercise perspective, the Sexual Six is going to be more enthusiastic about sport than the Self-Preservation Six.

Being the most ambiguous of the Enneagram types, Sixes may embrace a program one day, only to reject it the next, then feel bad for having done so and resume it later, only to have the pendulum swing back the other way and start all over again.

Exercise

Exercise is essential for releasing a Six's tension and anxiety. I've known Sixes become depressed overnight when they could not exercise. It's the shepherd that keeps the depression wolf at bay. What motivates them to exercise is the fear of what might happen if they don't. Most Sixes recognize the link between keeping fit and being healthier in old age. Often, though, they need to find this out for themselves, rather than be told what to do. It was only when a doctor was able to point out clearly to a Six and explain in great detail what gluten was doing to her body, how it was increasing her risk of coronary disease and Alzheimer's, that she finally started doing her own research, realizing that she needed to change her diet, if she was to live to a healthy old age.

For the "flight" type Six, fitness = security, a way to escape the demons they fear. As to what types of sports or exercise they choose, it will most likely be in the conventional arena—running, walking, team sports, cycling, golf, or working out at the gym. They enjoy routine and are happy to repeat the same workout for months, without seeming to get bored. This is good from the point of view of being regular exercise, but can mean they achieve a certain degree of fitness and won't push themselves beyond that. Here, their hard-working, dutiful nature comes to the fore, as they will stay with an exercise program, even if it is tedious and painful. Satisfaction comes with having exercised rather than the act of exercising itself. For example, imagine the swimmer who trains in the same pool daily for four hours a day every day, doing the same routine.

Unless, that is, the Six connects with the more Three aspect of themselves (the competitive side) and takes on fitness goals. Sixes are open to instruction from an authority, such as a personal trainer or coach whom they can rely on. They are happy to exercise alone,[13] but if they do choose a partner, it will be someone they trust and feel relaxed with. They can be very tolerant and supportive of a friend or team member who may not share their fitness level. I have a Six friend who walked loyally beside me, despite feeling frustrated at times that my pace was slower than hers. Sixes are looking for focus, peace, and security from the experience, so overly loud music, team members or coaches who let them down, or classes that are too full will annoy them. Ambiguous Sixes may one day be quiet and focused and on another, more open to conversation.

They see exercise as critical to their health and long-term safety but at the same time fear that too much exercise may result in injury. Unless they are counter-phobic types, you're unlikely to find them in high-risk sports, such as para-gliding or big wave surfing. They are too concerned about getting injured or what could go wrong.

It's my opinion based on an interview shortly before his death, that the now deceased legendary big wave rider Andy Irons was a counter-phobic Six. Irons was hugely courageous, but as he got older, his fear and vulnerability increased resulting in bipolar disorder, driving him to take increasing number of drugs and pills. It was just before a big competition that he was found dead in his hotel room.[14] (Note: it is not known if the death was accidental or not.)

Being organized means that Sixes won't leave things until the last minute when it comes to sporting events. As part of a team, they'll be the glue that holds things together. The go-to guy or gal. They have no problem scheduling daily exercise. Like Fives, they don't enjoy last-minute changes of plan. So if they normally have a run at lunchtime, and a boss tells them to attend a meeting during this time, they will find it hard not to feel annoyed with the disruption to their routine. As the Nike line goes, "Just do it!" Sixes view exercise as something that needs to be done and not necessarily as something to be enjoyed. They can view hiking with friends as leisure, while what they do in the gym is exercise.

My health insurance plan in South Africa offers an online fitness support group and benefits plan for members, where you accumulate points from exercise and healthy food purchasing that put you into various tiers with accompanying benefits, such as free smoothies, a sports watch, sports store discounts and so on. You receive points for carrying out various regular medical tests and points for sticking to weight-loss programs. You can even challenge friends and other members to various sporting and dietary goals. It's been hugely successful, and is the perfect program for Sixes who enjoy tracking achievements, optimizing their health, and feeling like they belong to a group.

Before a big sporting event, a Six's fear will emerge in sleepless nights pre-planning every eventuality. Will they injure themselves? What if they don't perform? What if their body doesn't respond properly? What if they let the team down? And so on. It can sometimes literally paralyze them—that feeling you may have had in a dream, where you want to run away but your legs become frozen.

After the event or practice, Sixes enjoy the camaraderie of a shared drink, coffee, or whatever the team or practice partners enjoy. It's the social reward for the hard work done. They'll enjoy reliving the event, sharing stories, and in an attempt to not stand out from the crowd and thus, be vulnerable to attack from envious others, they may play down their victories with self-deprecating jokes.

How to Inspire Sixes

Fear is the key issue with Sixes. To inspire them into a weight-loss program, they'll need to see that working out will give them more access to being with a group or crowd (safety in numbers). The team will support them. From a dietary perspective, being healthier means less likelihood of illness or disease (literally dis-ease), so they'll have less to fear healthwise. They will feel safer if they can run faster (flight) or be stronger (fight).

Levels of Health

Healthy

Healthy Sixes are warm, responsible, affectionate, and engaging. How this translates into eating patterns is that they have learnt to trust themselves and have self-confidence. This means that they have the self-worth to inspire the discipline to stick to an eating or exercise plan. They feel that they are worth it. Their sense of responsibility focuses not only on others but on being responsible to themselves to do what is best for them in terms of health.

While the odd fear may emerge, healthy Sixes are not anxiety-ridden. The self-confidence that has emerged now makes them excellent and loyal team leaders or captains, able to understand the hardship of the journey to succeed and able to lead by example. They have an inner knowing, which makes them an asset in a team where they can just "know" intuitively what the opposition team has planned.

They can laugh easily, often at themselves. They love asking questions of others: "What does your exercise routine entail?" "Tell me more about how you came to lose so much weight?" They are happy to share their success stories and tips with others who are trying to get healthier. They are genuinely interested in others and adopt a light, playful approach that endears them to colleagues and team mates.

Average

As the angst starts to emerge and dictate their lives, average Sixes start to doubt their decisions. What is genuine "knowing" and what is simply a confused voice in their heads? Which is the correct diet? Who is the authority they need to turn to for help? Their self-worth deteriorates, and although they may stick to an exercise routine or diet, it's more out of duty than wanting to be the best they can be. They may start doubting authority figures and rebel against them, which would include coaches, dietitians, doctors, and the like—people who may be genuinely trying to help them but whose motives now may be questioned. As they head closer to unhealthy levels of being, they may lash out at those who are trying to help them, seeing them one moment as help and the next as hindrance.

They become more anxious about their bodies and health. "Can my body really support me?" ("Do I have an illness?" "Am I having a heart attack or a panic attack?") Telling them not to worry isn't helpful. They need to feel that you have heard their angst.

Unhealthy

At this level, Sixes are often facing paranoia—here Sixes are the least able to handle stress of all types—seeing enemies where there are none. The very person trying to help them then becomes the target of their paranoid attacks. They may become obsessed with certain beliefs and those they see as gurus or systems: on the one hand wanting the security they seem to offer and on the other resenting and rebelling against it. They are afraid to lose this support, and yet seem to do everything to ensure that they will. Their worst fears start materializing. Highly skeptical, reactive, and cynical, they swing to extreme gullibility, pinning hope on charlatans and false promises, such as the "drink only coffee diet," expensive mail-order diet pills that promise miracle results, and gurus who convince them that their financial support and devotion will reward them with a slim and fit body (and enlightenment).

Self-destructive behavior sets in, and even though they know that their addictions are ruining their health and well-being, while they are doing them, the panic is kept momentarily at bay, hence the attraction to over-indulgence. It's the obese person, confined to a bed, who still orders in loads of sodas and grease-laden takeout food, even though they know it is life-threatening. Their inner guidance can no longer be trusted, just as they no longer trust themselves (or anyone else). They become prickly and oversensitive. Simply saying, "You've lost weight and look great in that dress" may be twisted so that they feel rather than having been given a compliment, you have in fact been belittling their efforts.

They may try to cover up their stress levels by appearing to be on top of things, because this makes them feel more adequate. "I've got this diet sorted," while the opposite may be true. Cutting off from their emotions they attempt to appear calm, but their mood swings and reactive behavior indicates otherwise.

They can swing from overeating to undereating, abuse booze, and feel unstable and un-grounded. Desperate and despairing, they search for security and become ever more reactive.

This can change if Sixes are prepared to work at recognizing when they are being reactive and swinging wildly like pendulums on adrenaline and so work toward calmness and steadfastness. Breathe deep. Let the anxiety out with each out-breath. Focus the "monkey mind" by being mindful. Recognize when you are projecting your fears onto others and seeing threats that are not real. You have a profound gift of inner knowing. Learn to trust it, so that you don't need to get validation from others. Be the courageous, grounded, compassionate person you are.

Summary

Sixes need to identify their fears and stress triggers if they are going to lose weight. If they don't become conscious of these, they will be tempted to revert to old patterns of eating when their security is shaken. Meditation, exercise, yoga, breathing exercises—whatever it takes to calm them and allows them to be okay with "being" rather than always "doing" will be hugely beneficial. It's important to note that in Sixes, stress triggers and depression typically start from outside sources, rather than, as is typical with Fours and Fives, an internal trigger. I've known Sixes turn depression around by acknowledging this outside source of stress and working to relieve the tension around the situation. It is best to seek help from a qualified professional.

Being able to see if you are a "fight" or "flight" Six also helps you become conscious of why you have either gained weight or are obsessed with keeping thin. Use your own inner guidance to determine which eating program to choose. Don't hand your power to others; learn from them, but don't make them gurus. Your natural desire to work hard, be committed, and follow routines is a huge advantage when it comes to weight-loss programs, but also take time to chill and smell the roses! Plus, if you're healthier, there is less need to worry about falling ill or health issues in general.

Type Seven
The Gallivanting Gourmet or the Discerning Diner

The Issue

Sevens seek instant gratification (from experiences, food, drink, or drugs). Food is an adventure, to be embraced with anticipation and excitement. Sevens want it all and go after what they want with immediacy and drive. Deep down, though, they fear deprivation. So they become acquisitive, constantly living in the future, planning what they desire to eat or do next. Activity then becomes a way to escape anxiety and fear, and the way they consume food becomes a way to stuff down concerns, rather than feel the pain of them.

Sevens hate to have any limits imposed upon them. Diets = limits, so it stands to reason that the idea does not appeal!

Overview of Type Seven

Sevens are fun to be with. They are charismatic, spontaneous, extroverted, and quick-thinking. Keeping up with them (or attempting to do so) can be exhausting!

Sevens are action-oriented optimists whose enthusiasm can be both charming and engaging. They are productive and have high levels of energy, while maintaining a curiosity about many things, which stimulates their creative, imaginative minds. They are busy, practical, and typically love a good party. Sevens are human *do*ings rather than human *be*ings. They are great to have around and can lift a whole room's emotion with their "*Always look on the bright side of life*" approach (from Monty Python's *The Life of Brian*).

They enjoy adventure, are thrill-seekers, and love planning the next outing or event. Typically, they are the types who having organized to have lunch at a certain place but will insist on stopping off along the way to a boutique winery, followed by sampling craft gin at a new distillery. They are freedom and future oriented and hate to be restricted by anyone or anything, so can sometimes appear as Peter Pans (men or women who won't grow up). They insist on keeping their options open. They are restless—like comets, they need to keep moving. They are both productive and prolific, preferring to see the overall vision of a project, rather than get stuck in the detail. To the extent to which they are healthy, they will fulfill their plans; the anacronym FOMO (Fear of Missing Out) was made for Sevens. They want to climb every mountain, taste every dish, visit every country, traverse every river ... there is no stopping them. Whereas Type Fours avoid people who they see as boring, Type Sevens avoid being bored by anything.

Sevens enjoy being the center of attention and are great raconteurs, often adding extra "flavor" to the story. They pick themselves up from failure quickly with no apparent long-term damage. You'll hear of them making fortunes, losing them, and making them again, all with apparent ease (think Virgin founder Richard Branson). Crypto-currency, such as Bitcoin, was made for Sevens!

When less healthy, Sevens are inclined to have great ideas but seldom bring them to fruition. In other words, they become scattered, flitting from one exciting idea to the next and not completing anything. They can begin to exaggerate, either to make the story funnier or to make their exploits appear larger, glossing over any obvious faults or failures. They can also limit the effects of their actions. "Yes, we did downscale, and there was some blood left on the walls, but we've moved on now" was how one Seven described letting go of many of his staff.

At average levels, Sevens may start to fly by the seat of their pants. Frustration and impatience arises, and they can become "Jacks of all trades but masters of none." It's as if there is a hot coal on their seat. They demand attention and lose inhibitions. "Have fun," they say. "Life is short."

As they become less healthy, the urge for stimulation can create total self-indulgence, agitation, and a hedonistic lifestyle, where life never moves out of the fast lane—escapists who can irresponsibly wreak havoc in the lives of others with their infantile and sometimes abusive behavior. Their schemes become wilder, their lives more debauched, and their personal handbrake doesn't function! Here, they can burn out and become addicted to risk and substances.

The choice for Sevens is to walk into the pain and work through it, or to carry on running until they exhaust themselves and often have to then confront it anyhow. If they choose the former, then they can satiate themselves with inner joy rather than outer experiences. They can affirm that their needs will be met on all levels. Like healthy Fives, they take time to not only observe but appreciatively smell the roses.

Career Choices

You'll find them as multi-taskers, entrepreneurs, in marketing, advertising, PR, as salespeople, travel writers, party planners, adventure guides, stuntmen, game wardens and park rangers, comedians, multi-business owners, artists, film makers, food critics, estate agents, professional athletes, restauranteurs, musicians, DJ's, gamblers—basically any career or activity that's seen as fun or that gets them out of a boring office routine and keeps them on the move. They also don't tend to enjoy being managed, so often end up creating their own businesses. They are unlikely to remain in the same field for their lifetimes and often pursue a wide variety of careers. Described by Russ Hudson as "Renaissance people",[1] they often have many talents and, with a risk-taking attitude, are not afraid to explore them.

Eating Triggers

Sevens are escapists, so when they feel emotional pain arising, they swing into planning mode, running away from these feelings (fear, anxiety, failure, being trapped or limited in any way, or actual physical pain or health issues). Part of the planning typically involves eating, drinking or drugs, or activities that are desired to create thrills. Food can also be a way to stimulate and create excitement, as, like gourmands, each taste brings with it a new experience.

Sevens want to avoid feeling deprived (and this includes food) or experience emotional pain in any shape or form. This is their wounding. They create a hedonistic busy lifestyle so as not to have to stop still, take a breath, and feel the resurgence of uncomfortable painful feelings.

As they become less emotionally healthy, they can move from feeling panicky into being out of control, swinging wildly from depression to manic behavior, where they'll eat, smoke, or drink anything, if it offers a glimmer of escapism.

How Sevens Approach Eating

You're on holiday. Fun time! Here you are at this tropical paradise, extra kilos and all, eyeing the tantalizing gourmet delights—all part of the Holiday Adventure Inclusive Package. You can learn to windsurf, scuba-dive, or go snorkeling. Parasailing's an option. River rafting holds possibilities. So does beach volleyball. Or lazing on the beach, cocktail in hand, while watching kite-boarders skim across the sea (you have a lesson booked for tomorrow).

Then there's the buffet, with its meters of seemingly endless food options. For starters, there's smoked salmon, as well as lobster, green bean, and radicchio salad, warm pancetta wrapped around brie with pesto dressing, phyllo cups with goat cheese and spring onions, maybe even fresh oysters or prawn cocktail, tuna terrine, stuffed green or plain kalamata olives, Thai shellfish broth, creamy mushroom soup. Then there's the main course and the inevitable Theme night area—anything from Creole to Cajun. Fish grilled to five-star perfection, chilli squid with lime dressing, the pasta area (your choice of carbonara, arrabiata, vongole or lasagne). The roast meat section—honey-roasted, juicy pork with apple sauce and crispy scratchings, legs of lamb with salted rosemary crust and mint sauce, roast beef with Yorkshire puddings, whole grain mustard, and to top it all, rich gravy. The vegetables—roast crispy potatoes, grilled brown mushrooms with Parmesan, fried cauliflower florets with herb salsa, baby marrow rolls stuffed with nutty wild rice, carrots in orange juice served with walnuts, green beans with anchovies and almonds... As well as the mountains of salad options, waiting to be covered with lashings of assorted dressings.

This is Seven heaven—all these choices. But as a Seven, you're already thinking about the desserts and cheese board.

Faced with a choice of food, a Seven will likely make life easier by choosing a bit of everything. That way, they'll neither miss out nor feel deprived in any way. There will also be no chance of having not eaten what the rest of the table decides is the best dish that day. The trouble is that, given this vast selection piled onto the plate, the tastes all seems to blend into each other—flavor mixing with flavor so that each dish loses rather than gains in appeal and the subtleties of taste and texture are lost in the gravy that ran onto everything. All this choice. All this food. And yet, afterwards the feeling that something is missing. This is the dilemma of the Seven.

Sevens Eating Out

Variety is the spice(y) lamb râgout of life for a Type Seven. They love choices and different experiences. Want to know about a new restaurant just opened in town? The latest delicatessen? Chances are your Seven friend will have already been and, if not, they'll have found out useful information about the place. Because Sevens (like Threes) are often First Adopters, not afraid to change, they are very likely to move beyond the tried and trusted to the new and exotic.

Connoisseurs who pride themselves on their food knowledge and sometimes even culinary expertise, Sevens would be even happier if they shared this love, surrounded by up-beat friends and a good bottle of cabernet (or three). They are fun-loving types who love to be with people, and if it's while experiencing new tastes and restaurants, even better. Hint: if you're opening a new restaurant, make sure you invite a whole bunch of Seven friends to spread the word afterwards.

Sevens are often the gourmands of the world, waxing lyrical (they like to talk!) on wine and food. They may be good chefs themselves in a creative or experimental way—they won't slavishly follow the recipe. Recipes are limiting; variations are exciting.

Claire has a Type Seven son who is 14 years old: "When he makes fudge, for instance, he will often change the recipe—add cherries, try making it chocolate rather than vanilla, and so on. He has mastered the basic recipe, and now he wants to explore new options." People who have set daily menus—Mondays = Spaghetti Bolognaise, Tuesdays = Vegetable Bake, and so on—would be unlikely to be Type Sevens.

One client reflected: "From the earliest days of my childhood, I remember being in the kitchen with my mother while she created diverse dishes. Cooking was an art form which she practiced with great love. She was, however, intolerably bored, she would tell us, with the preparation of mundane dishes. Mum never did boring. I'm afraid my rather basic tastes were a disappointment to her; cottage pie making did not hold the same allure as taking the basic dish and adapting it (sometimes it must be said with rather disastrous consequences)."

Sevens are also the most likely of all the personality types to try something new on the menu. Said one Seven: "The waiter was promoting a new vanilla-flavored wine. Although I knew it was an artificial flavor, I just wanted to see what it tasted like. My other wine-loving friends told me I was crazy—it was designed to make wine more palatable for teenagers—and it turned out they were right. The wine was foul, and I ended up leaving it. Still, I now know what artificially flavored wine is all about."

Sevens are often lavish and generous spenders, even if they can't really afford to be. The best wine and most exotic dishes at upmarket restaurants appeal to their consumerist nature. The relaxed French way of eating, though, where meals are long leisurely affairs, will not attract your average Seven, who will eat fast and then look for a distraction to "liven things up a bit!"

They also enjoy altering the dish to add excitement, such as, "I'll have the fish, but I'd like chopped chorizo in the sauce; it just gives it extra zing." They don't enjoy other people's food prescriptions for them, so ordering for them will not be appreciated (you've just limited their choice). Restaurants that offer variety with many taster portions will be preferred over a set menu.

They often order more than they can eat to avoid being stuck with one dish that's not appealing: "When we eat out, which we do often, I like to try out the menu. So we order several starters and main courses and then sample them all. I guess it's an expensive and wasteful thing to do, because we never finish the food, but it allows me to really get what a chef is on about in a restaurant." This from John, an entrepreneur who also has shares in a restaurant.

"One of the greatest experiences I had was to go with a top food critic to a restaurant where the chef specially prepared small helpings of his signature dishes and paired them each with great wine. Ten dishes in all, each prepared beautifully. It was an orgasmic experience," says a Seven advertising executive.

Because they are one of the more assertive personalities, Sevens are not afraid to send food back that they believe is not up to standard and can become quite demanding in restaurants if the service or food does not meet their high requirements. They pick up knowledge fast, so they may wax lyrical and enthusiastically about food varieties and wine types, which may irritate those who have really mastered the subject (like Fives), if that was their interest. It's not that a Seven is a know-it-all; rather, they are okay with the idea that some knowledge gives them the right to discuss issues; they don't have to have mastered the subject.

Optimistic Sevens will tend to take the best aspects of the evening and focus on those: "Okay, the food wasn't great and it was overpriced, but the band was fun, don't you think?" is typical of a Seven's take on what others may describe as a disappointing evening. A bad dining experience will quickly be overlooked in the quest for something new and better.

Sevens, and Nines, would be the most likely Enneagram type to arrive late. Nines because they prioritized incorrectly, Sevens because this function was on a long list of social activities planned for the evening. Or on the way to the restaurant, a Seven may have made plans to drop off an item borrowed from a friend, see a client, then stop to meet a colleague for a drink. Not allowing enough time for each task has now seen the Seven arrive late. However, with their customary charismatic charm, they will apologize (possibly) and make light of it. If present company is not upbeat enough, they'll quickly move on.

They are, as mentioned, future oriented (together with Fives and Sixes). With a Seven, the anticipation of a meal (future thinking) of food and drink, going to a restaurant, and so on is very important.

"At dinner, I'll order the nachos starter and then maybe do the ribs (they do those so well at El Macho's), followed by the brownies…"

"When I know we are going to a new restaurant, I often Google the menu, so that I can consider my menu choice. I may not necessarily stick to it, but I enjoy just thinking about and planning my meal."

Russ Hudson and the late Don Riso refer to this anticipation of a meal or experience as the Chocolate Syndrome: anticipation, craving, and excess.[2]

Sevens can encourage others to go to places they would not normally go. "Our 50-something book club was persuaded by a Seven to head to a burger bar where the male waiters were all gorgeous and didn't wear shirts. It was a wild evening which, if it hadn't been planned for us, would never have happened," one woman reflects.

Sandra, a graphic designer, explains: "When I worked out of town, it was a 10-minute walk to the nearest café. I used to plan my day not on my work schedule but on an eating schedule: 11:00 meant a walk to get a packet of chips, 13:00 meant a walk to get a yogurt and an apple, and so on. What I was eating then wasn't a lot really, or particularly unhealthy, and I wasn't at all overweight, but my constant focus on the food as a reward and anticipating it, was not healthy. It also broke up the day into bits, making my restlessness less problematic."

Being generous, Sevens will often pick up the tab, even if they really can't afford to do so. While other types may be carefully dividing the bill according to what each person ate and drank, the Seven will see this as boring and nit-picking.

Sevens Entertaining at Home

It's 6:15 p.m., and the guests are due in less than an hour. The Seven has just returned from the shops, purchasing food for the evening (when the going gets tough, the tough go shopping!). They haven't decided exactly what they'll be serving other than lamb. They're late because a few extra chores and a call planning tomorrow's events took longer than expected. But our Seven is "on it." *Ready, Steady, Cook*,[3] here our Seven comes! They find measuring and weighing boring, so they'll toss in a bit of this and that with flare.

Sevens can be great cooks, enjoying lavish meals shared with exotic friends. In the Danish film, *Babette's Feast* (a cult classic for foodies), set in a small coastal fishing village, Babette goes to great lengths to source exotic foodstuffs from Paris to cook a magnificent meal for the locals. They fail to appreciate the effort and expense that has gone into the preparations—an eight-course meal lovingly prepared—when soup and bread would have sufficed. This abundance is very much part of a Seven. Much of the meal may have been purchased from various delicatessens and specialist stores, so the actual preparation is more of a setting out than cooking from scratch. What they love is bringing some new dish or drink to the table, which they can wax lyrical about to their guests, or describe the specialist store where it was purchased.

A traditional "meat and two veg" meal simply won't work—it's way too boring. Presentation is very important, so they'll make the effort to have just the right stylish plates and boards to lay out their food.

You would imagine that Sevens would enjoy learning something new, but it's not so. Learning is confining, tedious, and wastes too much time. New experiences in food, yes; cooking classes that last longer than a fun evening with friends, no.

Sevens want their guests to have as much fun as they intend having, so no expense will be spared. They are normally not particularly neat, preferring stylish comfort over order. Their spaces often look like they've just had a party or are gearing up for the next one. Touches of bright color will often abound, trendy music will blare, and exotic cocktails will flow freely.

Food Choices

For Sevens, shopping for food is a potential adventure. They'll traipse around the countryside to find just this wine or that truffle oil. They enjoy knowing a lot about food and each product. If they are wealthy, this exploration can cross continents. The proviso, though, is that the food must look good, so packaging is important. Take two salamis and hand-wrap one in brown paper with a rustic string and well-designed logo and it will win out every time over a commercially sealed plastic wrap (in this, they can resemble Type Fours).

Like Type Threes, Sevens can also be fast-food junkies. Being constantly on the go, they may not allow themselves the time to sit down and leisurely eat a meal; heading for a drive-through for takeout may make perfect sense. That way they can satisfy their hunger while driving *and* talking on the cell phone.

Because of their high-energy levels, many Sevens burn up their calorie intake very quickly, while some may become so preoccupied with the new exciting turn of events with their latest project that the idea of food disappears in order to accommodate other excitement and other ways (apart from eating) to fend off boredom. Being "thinking" types they can lose connection with their body and their body's needs.

Should they decide to become vegetarians or vegans, it will most likely be because it's the latest fad way of eating and switching will provide more food choices. If they lean heavily toward a Type Six, then like Sixes, they may become vegetarian out of sympathy for the animals.

They approach life and food by trial and error (*I'll try this. If I don't like it, then I'll try something else. Even if it's not what I really want, it'll shift the focus away from what I really crave emotionally (but may be unaware of) to what fulfils me now. Hmmm, what shall I have? Trifle, ice cream, cheesecake, or an éclair?*). The dessert trolley offers huge potential, so just to be sure they don't miss out, they'll have a bit of everything. They have lost that deep connection to their intuitive selves that would have guided them to healthier options.

Remember the joke about the people on the *Titanic* who decided not to have dessert that fateful night? The point being they missed the opportunity, held themselves back, and to what end? They died unfulfilled—not a pleasant prospect for a Seven.

For a Seven, life is too short to put limits on oneself. This applies to eating. Whereas a Type One may pride themselves on being disciplined and avoiding fattening foods, a Seven will revel in the enjoyment of doing just the opposite and be damned with the consequences. A wonderful slice of cheesecake affirms to the Seven the goodness of life and overrides the niggling feeling that this may not be doing their cholesterol level or waistline any good. With Sevens life is full of so much to be experienced that it can feel exhausting at times. Just how many places are there to eat out? How many options to choose from on each menu?

How many distractions to follow? This vast amount of opportunity, while exciting, can never be fully experienced, so the Seven can never feel completely fulfilled.

Sevens typically love to shop up a storm! This includes shopping for food and wine. They are any advertiser's dream, as all you have to do is dangle the word "new" in front of them and they will just have to try it. They may only be buying a meal for one, but chances are they'll emerge from the store with several options. They are food and wine snobs, so in-store brands won't work for them. They'll toss way too much into their shopping cart in their gregarious, generous way.

Chatting to the owner of the *fromagerie* about the origins of each of the cheeses (as a Five might do— this is because Sevens move toward Fives on the Enneagram) is an enjoyable pastime for the Seven, and any interesting stories discovered will be told later at dinner. Their impulsive buying leads them to exotic items—pâtés, imported delicacies, desserts, and so on—but steers clear of bland foods such as vegetables or lentils.

Sevens snack mindlessly when they are bored—salty or sweet, whatever distracts them from the anxiety that arises if nothing is planned for later.

What You May Not See

"How are you," I asked a Seven. "Fab! Great! All good!" came the standard reply. Sevens don't want anyone to see the side of them that is depressed, lonely, and unhappy. A Seven friend's husband and two children were attacked by two knife-wielding thugs. They managed to escape unharmed, but it was a terrifying situation. The standard response to my enquiry as to the family's well-being was "Fab!" When I suggested trauma counseling for the girls and their father, the mother wouldn't hear of it. "They're fine. All good."

Sevens don't want you to see them the morning after the party, when their apartment is trashed, their Botox needs attention, their lover has left them for another, and they are eyeing the cocaine stash. When they do appear to face the world, hyped up on anything from drugs to painkillers, (unhealthy Type Seven), the sadness will be masked by a pseudo positivity, that, as they disintegrate, becomes increasingly more vulnerable.

Not wanting to go there, they will be planning activities to propel them into a busy happy place. When I probed one Seven about how they experience their feelings of sadness, they said to me: "I just have a cup of tea and grab a book, or else I head to the ocean to ride some waves. That sorts things out. I just don't understand depression."

How They View Their Bodies

One problem with the busyness that Sevens create in their lives is that they are so busy that they can neglect to take care of their physical needs. They may skip meals, only to gorge later on unhealthy snacks.

A Seven said to me: "I realized that I was going through the day seldom, if ever, getting around to drinking any water, which is bland and boring. Dehydration, though, wasn't good for my health. I always just wanted to finish this or do that first. When evening came, I sat down for a drink and, being very thirsty, gulped the alcohol. Now I've realized that I don't drink enough water, I try to say to myself one glass of water before each cup of coffee or glass of wine. It's helped hugely."

Sevens want their bodies to reflect their desire to be attractive, which will enhance their appeal and allow them to be part of the "in" crowd and look cool. When their body threatens to let them down, and they feel themselves to be overweight or unattractive, their bodies can become the enemy, thwarting their potential fun. They are drawn to cosmetic surgery as a quick-fix solution to what they see as physical flaws. They may then go to extremes to recreate the beauty they once had, or believe they need to have, to still be attractive. Cosmetic surgery itself can become an addiction.

Not wanting to dwell on anything they see as being negative or painful, Sevens can ignore major health warnings. They'll mean to go to the doctor for a check-up regarding that lump, but delay going or "forget" appointments, rather than run the risk of confronting what could be a serious issue. They often leave it too late, when early intervention could have averted the problem.

As they get older, their concern about their health increases, and they often hone in on any slight discomfort. They are basically more afraid than normal of being trapped in bodies that don't allow free movement or that are riddled with pain. Creating adventures and distractions is a way of avoiding this rising fear. The most terrifying experience for a Seven friend was having a back operation that required lying flat for two weeks, completely reliant on nurses for everything. Not a pleasant prospect for anyone, but to a Seven, terrifying. When life is only enjoyed when you are experiencing diversity and stimulation, this situation would be absolute torture.

Addictions

Sevens have addictive personalities.[4] They feel a constant need to stay up and "on top of their game." Stimulants will attract them, rather than antidepressants or dope, and will include caffeine, amphetamines, ecstasy, alcohol, sugar, cocaine—anything that will give them an emotional lift. Constant working and partying is unsustainable, so they need pick-me-up drugs to continue to stay high, rather than risk feeling low.

Fashion is another potentially fun experience. They quickly get bored with their current wardrobe and enjoy acquiring new outfits. They keep abreast of the latest trends. Bright, bold, exciting, and "out-there" appeals to them. Like Imelda Marcos and her 1,220-plus pairs of shoes, purchasing can become an addiction.

The deep-seated fear and anxiety (often not visible to those around them or even themselves) causes stress in the Seven, which is relieved by eating. However, the relief is only temporary, until the stress builds up again. The eating or drinking or substance addictions are a way to suppress emotions and release tension, providing the escapism that Sevens love. The greater the stress, the greater the desire to consume whatever is the Sevens' addiction.

When stressed, Sevens can also start to behave like unhealthy Ones, feeling the need to educate and judge others about their bad eating habits while covertly eating in an unhealthy manner themselves—the dietitian who binges would be an example. They may use the energy of their One influence to try hard to rein in their appetite and impose greater self-control, but because of their intense dislike of being restricted or trapped into a regime, they will eventually rebel and succumb to their appetite's desires. Like unhealthy Ones, this rebellion usually results in a full-scale binge of some sort, with the accompanying aftermath of guilt and shame.

The constant desire to remain up and engaging in fun experiences means that Sevens are seldom present, because everything seems more fun somewhere else. They become slaves to their own needs to not miss out and to keep searching for the new best thing.

Being part of the hip, happening crowd can become something of an addiction. They can develop fascinations with certain people, only to drop them and move on when a more exciting prospect appears. Ever been at a party chatting to someone, when you are aware they are not listening to you but looking to see what other guests have arrived who would be more entertaining? This addiction to not being present but watchful for a more exciting future can make Sevens appear shallow.

Going into any form of rehabilitation program is extremely unappealing to a Seven; the very nature of the 12-Step program for addiction recovery is limitation, and it will feel slow and often unbearable to a Seven, who has spent their life running away from deprivation. Feeling trapped, Sevens will seek freedom by heading back to their "fun" addictions. Everyone else will appear boring in the program. "Come on, have some fun. You only live once" will be the language they will use to persuade others to head off the rails and party with them.

Childhood

Food is associated with nurturing. The nurturer is in most cases, but not always, the mother. If the Seven felt or experienced being disconnected to the main nurturing figure, or if the nurturance received was experienced as being inconsistent or unreliable, then the child learns to look for nurturing outside their principal nurturing relationship. This causes the child to become fearful of being deprived or anxious when limitations are placed on nurturing. Rather than experience the pain of the feeling of loss, Sevens learn distraction as a means of avoidance of painful feelings.[5] To work through these feelings of not having their emotional needs met, Sevens may have transferred their unmet needs to exterior objects, which are controllable by them. As a young child, this could be a toy and later can become food, other objects, or substances.

The word "gluttony" is associated with Sevens and naturally includes desire for food and alcohol but also encompasses all experiences.[6] Sevens at an early age attempt to nurture themselves (*If I can't have what I want, I'll go out and get it myself*).

One Seven described the separation from her mother like this: "Before and during my conception, my father was having an affair. My mother was understandably very upset and depressed about the situation. I guess, although she loved me, the focus of her attention was on her unmet needs, rather than mine."

Sevens may also have experienced a childhood history where scarcity was an issue, either through poverty or possibly through a cautious parent with a tight budget. Whatever the cause, the result was a child who wanted to avoid the feeling of "not enough" ever again—Oliver Twist's begging, "Please, sir, can I have some more?" and being refused.

This fear of lack then is overcome by stocking up as much as possible, while it's available (like many Fives), because the thinking is *What if it's not there later when I am actually hungry?* Add to this the Seven's desire for stimulation and experience and you get *I want to experience all the options in case the opportunity passes me by.* They have developed a fear of not having their needs met. They create ways to divert their fears into activities. Like a mouse on a treadmill they keep on the move, fearing that if the treadmill stops they will have to confront uncomfortable fears and feelings.

One Seven's parents had lived through two world wars and were consequently very "careful" when it came to food. Used to war rations, they insisted on their children eating a slice of bread before a meal to fill them up before the "better" food appeared.

"Meals were calculated with precision: Five people = five chops, five baked potatoes, and so on," said the Seven.

If a guest stopped by for dinner unexpectedly, it was usually the Seven's mother who claimed that she wasn't hungry, so the guest could eat.

"When I married, I went overboard entertaining generously by making far too much choice available and preparing way too much food," she explained. "I never wanted my guests or family to feel limited, as I had done."

Diets for Sevens

To a Seven, the world may feel like their oyster, but they may not know when to stop eating them ("Don't try to restrict me!").

The Rebel archetype is alive and well in the psyche of a Seven with a Six wing. Mention dieting and, while at first a Seven may seem to comply, it won't be long before they find the whole process tedious and can't resist the temptation to try something more exciting than what has been specified. Diets are way too limiting and simply no fun! ("Life is too short to not have what you enjoy!")

The fear of deprivation makes Sevens the least likely to stick to any form of diet, because diets = deprivation. It's easier for a Seven to participate in exercise to work off the weight than it is for them to cut down on what and how much they eat.

Dietitians, doctors, and health clinics are perceived as being major limiting factors—boring, overbearing people who evoke the memory of parents who deprived them of their foremost need. That's painful to feel, and Sevens don't want to feel pain at any cost. Consulting health professionals for weight loss, becomes an uncomfortable experience they would rather avoid.

To divert the dietitian's attention away from the fact that the Seven has not stuck to their intended diet, they may switch on the charm and try to rationalize their actions.

"I went to a diet club with the intention of following the program. Naturally it didn't happen, so instead of confronting the issue of why within myself, I turned the whole process of weighing and measuring into a charming joke. I was full of lengthy explanations, as to why I had not complied. Any attempt by the supervisor to criticize my actions was met either with humor to deflect the problem, or lengthy stories about the nature of dieting itself, snippets of research, food intolerances, or anything rather than actually deal with the issue at hand: I simply wasn't following the program."

In this way, they attempt to make the dietitian their buddy, and buddies don't limit their friend's fun.

A very ill and obese Seven told me: "I have quite a few cancerous tumors—two quite large ones near my liver. I have opted not to have chemo, so the oncologist has me on this strict diet. In the morning, I have to drink this whole concoction of healthy things, but in the evening I drink wine, and lots of it!"

This is a typical response from a Seven. Weighing, measuring, lack of variety, or limiting intake won't work. The diet needs to be entertaining.

In their attempts to rein in their wayward eating ways, a Seven may be in denial that there is a weight problem at all, even if physicians have warned them of the negative effect extra weight is having on their body. As noted above, diets that involve limiting foods or keep track of details like weekly weigh-ins or keeping a food journal are not going to work. There are far more interesting things to do than stopping to record how many cookies they are sneaking or how many times they've strayed from their eating plan. They can be glib and clever in their approach, though. They may have been caught red-handed, spoon in the Double Cream Rocky Road ice cream, but they will quickly turn the tables on whoever found them out, making them feel like a party pooper and wrong for calling them out.

At parties, they may snack unconsciously and not be aware of how many canapes they have consumed. This can be a dangerous time for a dieter, particularly if alcohol is added to the mix, because with a couple of drinks under their belt, they are likely to cross the line they have set for themselves, and all restraint goes out the window. Sevens have an issue with fear. Alcohol and drugs quells this fear, which is what makes them so appealing, because behind this pathologically upbeat Seven, is a frightened, anxious child.

Ask a Seven "What's eating away at you?" and they will run for the hills! Introspection is not appealing, so they will be loath to go to therapy to work on their issues.

The emotions of Sevens tend to be projected outward rather than felt internally. When a painful emotion starts welling up inside, the feeling is quickly diverted to a new experience, which often involves food or drink. Food appears to create happiness and a diversion from less comfortable feelings.

Use the word "discipline" or "diet," and the Seven will head for the hills; use the words "exciting new lifestyle change," though, and you'll get their attention. Dietitians often meet with resistance from Sevens, who do not want to listen to others, particularly anyone trying to restrict them in any way; rather, they want to experience things for themselves.

"I have been sent to three different dietitians by three different doctors, all concerned about my weight and the health threats it poses (Type 2 diabetes runs in my family). I realized that I needed to lose weight and sat patiently through all the information and went off and really did try for a few days. However, this other part of myself would well up and say, 'What's the point. Why restrict yourself today when a bus could end your life tomorrow?' When it came to weighing day, I used my wit to win the dietitians over, until we moved beyond the topic of food and my failure to adhere to the diet. At one clinic, I remember they even called in one of the 'heavies' (excuse the pun) to give me a lecture. It didn't work, though. The shame quickly passed. I wanted to lose the weight but wasn't prepared to be restricted or limited. I thought just spending the money would make me feel bad and make me comply, but it didn't. The voice saying 'What the hell' was stronger."

Because of this need to feel full (full-filled) and the pace at which they often eat, Sevens often consume more than they need. The appetite rules the head long before the appestat has time to kick in. But it's not just a physical appetite, or the simple need for nourishment, but an appetite for life itself: do, experience, take as much in as possible, that way you'll miss out on nothing ("The more I eat, the less fear I have of not really living").

Try:

- Taking half the amount of food each mouthful.

- Chewing food at least 20 times before swallowing.

- Taking double the amount of time to complete a meal and focus on the food itself. As you eat more slowly, you'll find that you start noticing subtleties in the taste and texture of the food that you've probably overlooked.

- Avoiding distractions such as TV, answering emails, or working simultaneously on the computer.

- Dishing up half the normal amount of food, with the understanding that you can dish up the second part later after a 10-minute break, should you desire.

- Taking time to savor the subtle taste of each mouthful. Taste what it is you have now on the plate, rather than chase an escapist desire.

- Enjoying simple foods—the crisp crunch of a fresh carrot, the subtle taste of a cucumber stick, the effect that a piece of basil leaf has on a ripe tomato slice...

- Sharing the feeling of being afraid with a partner or close friend—not with the expectation that they should "heal" the feeling but simply to give you space to feel and acknowledge the fear.

- Asking yourself, when you are bored, what emotions you are not wanting to feel or may want to avoid. Let yourself feel this emotion. By feeling it, you can heal it.

- Moving into gratitude for the food you have in front of you. For the people who worked hard to bring you this experience.

Eating Too Fast

Whereas a Two might eat too quickly because they feel ashamed of their eating habits and want the experience to be over, a Seven may eat too quickly because they are either afraid of missing something or alternatively because they want to take in as much as possible, before moving on to the next course/experience.

A student who was a Seven said: "I guess if I were to pinpoint a time when I started picking up weight, it was when, after studying, I was doing some traveling and took a temporary job at a London pub. Until then I'd been very thin. At the pub, though, there were all these different menu options to choose from, none of them healthy. After traveling and living off $5 a day, free food was a most welcome job perk, even though it was stodgy, overcooked, and often fried in lots of oil. Chips, bangers, pies, mushy peas—you get the idea. After a four-hour shift, I was ravenous and started helping myself to a bit of everything. It tasted so good after watching every one of the customers eat and not being able to do so myself (deprivation). We only had a short time to eat before cleaning up the pub and knocking off. Other staff got impatient if you hung around too long, so it was all about eating lots and fast." This is typical of a Seven's thinking.

Another Seven told me: "I started out too quickly, I guess, when I had kids. Life was so hectic, trying to work from home and do nappies and so on, so meals were always eaten on the trot, supplemented by whatever the toddlers left. A cheese-and-ham sandwich eaten while answering emails or feeding a two-year-old, a few biscuits stuffed into my mouth while hanging the washing. It was all about having no time to nurture myself and all about nurturing others. I could not believe it when my husband started working from home, how much effort he would put into making his lunch—nifty salads, healthy soups. He didn't seem to feel the pressure to rush the preparation the way I did.

"Needless to say, with each child I put on more weight and became more resentful at not giving myself time to make healthy food and sit down to eat. It was always rush, rush. Silly, really, now that I look back on it—the extra half-hour to prepare and eat seemed so impossible to find. I've never lost that gulp-down food habit, though. I am always conscious that others are only halfway through their meals while I've finished mine. I've read that this doesn't allow one's appestat to check in, so you eat more than you really need, which figures."

The appestat is a hypothetical region of the brain, most likely located in the hypothalamus or near the pituitary gland. Its function is to help regulate the appetite. If you are aware of your body, you will listen to your body's feeling of being full and stop eating. When functioning optimally, the appestat, together with the adipostat (believed to be a series of hormonal outputs), sends a message to the brain when you're full. Yet they can be easily overridden, particularly in the case of people who eat too quickly. It takes approximately 20 minutes for the brain or neurotransmitters from the brain to communicate and register a feeling of fullness. By eating too fast, you've finished a whole lot more food than you actually need before this message can come into play. Even if you do eat fast, eat less, and although you initially may still feel hungry after a meal, when your appestat does kick in, you'll feel full. If you feel full before 20 minutes has passed, it's a sure indication that you've bitten off way more food than you need to chew.

Because they live in anticipation, Sevens can be eating one dish whilst already imagining eating the next and as a result not truly enjoying either. The appetite rules the head. It is an appetite for life itself: do, experience, take as much in as possible; that way you'll miss out on nothing.

Exercise

Throughout the day, Sevens will be fuelling their anxiety, resulting in a build-up of stress levels. Because they are unable to really acknowledge how they are feeling, they are often in denial that they are stressed. A large meal topped off with several large glasses of tipple becomes their way of suppressing rather than expressing this stress/fear. It goes under the banner of "I've worked really hard today so I deserve a little fun/indulgent food/drink." It can be extremely helpful for Sevens to take this stress and channel it into challenging exercise.

Sevens can be motivated to exercise if they understand that poor health may lead them into pain and deprivation; however, fear is never an ideal or long-term motivator. Exercise can be painful, and as we know pain is feared by Type Sevens, so exercise that doesn't involve too much pain or where the excitement overrides the pain, will be more successful.

They have far more self-confidence than the other types (except for Type Eight), so no matter what their body shape, they are usually not concerned with going to the gym. They want to look cool and trendy, but being "a bit" overweight won't detract from this in their minds. They live in the future, so past failures are quickly glossed over and forgotten. If they have lost an important match, they bounce back sooner than other types. Use your Seven love of adventure and experience to work with your body in a positive manner. Do an exciting sport. I'm not necessarily talking about base jumping but something that you enjoy and find stimulating. Riding a wave has more thrills, variations, and entertainment value than, say, weightlifting.

Sports that are not dully repetitive, such as board-sailing, stand-up paddle-boarding, surfing, hiking Mount Everest, or mountain biking, involve constant new challenges and an adrenaline rush, which Sevens enjoy.

"I never really regarded surf-sailing as exercise," one Seven told me. "Exercise to me = boredom and repetition. With surf-sailing, each new wave ride was a new challenge—something to be mastered. I was super-thin then but did it for the fun rather than to maintain weight. I just loved it. When I stopped because I couldn't take the time out, with a young family, I really missed it and ended up putting on kilos."

Through this type of activity, Sevens can feel their fear, even if it's now symbolized in a wave, steep mountain, and so on. This releases it, stress levels drop, and the need to overeat or drink diminishes.

It takes repetition and practice to excel in a sport. This is problematic for a Seven, who can find training limiting and boring. They often leave sports in which they show promise, simply because they are looking for greater stimulation.

In team sports, the party after the win, or the team vibe on the way to an event, is as important, if not more so, than the actual game. They love socializing with the team and being one of the gals or guys. Sport that offers travel opportunities is even better. Their naturally upbeat nature makes them great for team morale and motivation. They also love to win and are fierce competitors, throwing everything behind whatever sport it is in order to take home the trophy. But if the sport starts feeling repetitive, they will leave, even if they are enjoying success.

This desire to win at all costs means that, like Threes, they are very susceptible to taking performance-enhancing drugs. The Three wants the approval of winning and feeling the best, while the Seven wants the thrill of winning against the odds. It's the excitement of winning that propels them onto the next challenge. Threes don't mind the hard win—they'll train as long and as hard as it takes. Sevens want the easy win.

How to Inspire Sevens

I drove past a car today with a bumper sticker emblazoned with the words "PARTY YOUR WEIGHT AWAY." The idea was to dance, and in doing so, the pounds would fall away and you'd get fit. Every passing Seven would be attracted to this. To get Sevens onboard requires making things more fun.

But be careful that in order to avoid the pain they might feel about their weight, Sevens don't end up entertaining you to the point that you never get them to really own or delve into the issue, so it remains the literal elephant in the room, clouded by fun stories and upbeat humor. They will zone out if things get too heavy or boring, so you need to keep things vibey. They need to understand that by working on themselves, they will *be* more, feel more, and enjoy greater depth of experience;[7] that exploring their inner world is where the real juice is to be found and not in outside experiences. Doing so will create the freedom and real joy they desire. Having a healthier, more mobile physique is a big step toward this, and a way of helping to ensure they aren't trapped in the pain and ill health of their physical selves.

Levels of Health

Healthy

As they move toward becoming healthy, Sevens become more focused and less scattered. Task planning becomes task completion. Their minds and eating habits slow down. They can make more conscious food choices. The endless need for fulfilment (*full-fill me*) is replaced with an ability to slow down and savor each mouthful, rather than focusing on imagining what the next course will taste like. Fulfilment then is not a goal but a state of being. They can confront the fears and emotions they have been running from and work through them, without using food as a crutch. Sevens can now examine their genuine needs and seek to satisfy these. They learn self-restraint and contentment. They have realized that no amount of chocolate cake can satiate their deep inner longing for relationship with themselves.

Their minds are receptive. At this higher level of consciousness, Sevens can be happy with very little because they trust that their needs will be met. They are like Buddhist monks who walk from village to village with only the clothes they wear and a begging bowl for food. With all the baggage of their emotional lives left behind, emotionally healthy Sevens are no longer ruled by their fear of deprivation and pain. They truly feel joy in the experience of the present moment and are grateful for all that is.

Average

Living in the future is very much part of the less healthy and average Seven's perspective on life. So even while eating pizza the Seven is not present, enjoying each cheesy mouthful; rather, they are ahead of the game, projected into the future and the potential that the chocolate fudge sundae could hold.

If we aren't present we can never really enjoy life, because we are either focusing on the shame and regret of the past or projecting ourselves into a fearful future that rarely occurs the way we expect it to. Buddhists sometimes refer to this state of mind as being like a "hungry worm." The Seven then is in a no-win situation. The craving, followed by the fulfilment of that craving, leads only to more craving, because the mind is already headed into the expectation of the more rewarding experience in the future. Gluttony cannot be satiated.

The enjoyment of the food is thus decreased, because they can't fully appreciate what they are eating now. As they become unhealthier, they can turn greedy and life becomes all about selfishly gratifying their own needs whilst ignoring the needs of others. Food "fixes" satisfy their inner cravings momentarily, so they become less discriminating about food choices. They may also deny the extent of their weight problem, describing obesity as "carrying a few extra pounds."

The anticipation of the meal has become greater than the actual experience of eating and enjoying it. This can apply to places as well as food. If I'm sitting at a quaint French restaurant in my local town, I may be fantasizing about eating the meal at a restaurant I've read about in France. Even more tantalizing experiences still await me. So I become the hungry worm, never enjoying the present meal but always anticipating better meals or courses.

As one Seven put it: "If I'd ordered the beef, my partner's lamb looks a better option. The more I disintegrate, the greater my need becomes for new foodie experiences. I now crave only a certain type of coffee and will drive miles to have some. I only want a particular exclusive wine—nothing else is good enough; yet even when I'm drinking it, I am already planning the aperitif."

Unhealthy

The more they experienced a traumatic or unstable childhood, the greater the chances that a Seven will experience a feeling of emotional emptiness.

Life then becomes about constantly looking for something to fill the gap.

At their unhealthier emotional levels (which often translate into physical ill health), Sevens will show little restraint, and instant gratification rules. Their addiction to unhealthy food and drinks will lead them to overindulge in alcohol, sodas, coffee, cakes, and so on. Food becomes an addiction to help stave off their worries and fears.

Even when warned by health professionals about their unhealthy life style and eating patterns, they are unlikely to take heed, feeling that such warnings merely restrict their right to enjoyment and having fun. They may also do their own personal research to counteract these findings. For instance, Paul's reaction to the results of a blood test that revealed too much alcohol in his blood was to research the antibiotics he was on and find that one of the related side effects was a possibility of an inaccurate blood count reading. Using this information, he discounted the results (and his own alcohol intake).

While change is easier to deal with for a Seven than most other types, if it is perceived to involve diet, or food deprivation on some level, chances are they will resist healthier options and despite the negative and possibly even serious health effects of their eating habits, choose to enjoy today what could destroy them tomorrow. Its "eat, drink, and be merry for tomorrow we die" for Sevens.

As they become unhealthier, Sevens are unable to say no to themselves and can become gluttons indulging in all forms of excess, from food to drugs to drinking, habits that escalate as they further deteriorate into the lower unhealthy levels. Here, they can become even more self-destructive, impulsive, undisciplined, and rebellious—none of which are great characteristics for sticking to a controlled way of eating. They can be indiscriminate in their choices and insensitive to the needs of others ("I like pasta, so that's what we are having. If your wheat intolerance is a problem, then make your own supper"). An example would be that of a morbidly obese man I knew. He refused to change his eating patterns, even when it became clear that his life was at stake. His fear of being deprived was far stronger than his fear of dying.

The very pain and deprivation Sevens seek to avoid, they can, through their recklessness, impose on others.

If Sevens can see where this destructive behavior is headed, they can start to climb back up the ladder to health. They need to truly understand that no amount of external experience is going to give them the long-term satisfaction and fulfilment they desire. True joy comes from within and radiates into the loving experience of the present. No amount of planning can achieve this. Savoring will be their savior. Authentic living becomes the vast and plentiful banquet of life.

Summary

Sevens need to bring more focused attention to all they do and this includes their eating and exercise habits. They need to confront their fears and work through them, so that they can assimilate experiences, rather than use food/drink to suppress the fear. If not addressed they will continue to crave and consume.

When they become healthier, they learn to practice restraint without feeling deprived, because they know on a deep level what will truly fulfil them. Their often irresponsible Peter Pan self matures emotionally so that they can be honest with themselves. Gratitude and joy replace inner craving, irresponsibility, and the fear of being deprived, because they intuitively know their worth and that their needs will be met. Authentic happiness is their reward.

Type Eight
The Binging Bully or the Forgiving Feaster

The Issue

In historical cartoons, the boss is often characterized as being a large person. Not that all Type Eights are large but they may have big chests, so-called "heavyweights" who puff themselves out to appear important. Seeking to hide their vulnerable side, they appear strong and confident. They are lusty creatures, going after what they want with drive and passion, and this includes what they eat. And with no limitations! This does not bode well for weight-loss regimes.

Overview of Type Eight

Type Eights have larger-than-life personalities. When an Eight walks into the room, you have the immediate feeling that they are in charge. "Don't mess with me," they seem to say. Another favorite saying might be, "When the going gets tough, the tough get going!" They literally throw their weight around. Heavy hitters and heavy weights—in a business sense. They make things happen and encourage others to do the same. They take risks, enjoying the challenge and the sweetness of success. They are strong (often physically) and passionate about life, with a lusty "go get it" attitude. This lust for life translates into an immediacy when it comes to desiring something or someone.

They are resourceful and independent and enjoy being the boss rather than the employee. They are straight talkers and don't respect those who can't match their desire to confront (they enjoy confrontation).

These are big-hearted people. They can be both protective of those they see as being in their inner circle and vengeful toward anyone they see as having threatened them or anyone close to them. They want freedom for themselves and fear being controlled or taken advantage of by anyone else (yet paradoxically, can do just that to others). They hate feeling vulnerable in any way.

They are assertive and action-oriented and enjoy the competition that occurs between rival companies (as long as they win in the end!). To this end they are fierce opposition, yet when healthy, want to be seen as someone to be respected and whose word can be counted upon. They can be willful and tend to dominate others, sometimes seeing those around them as extensions of themselves, without their own desires, wishes or needs. The counter-phobic Eight, however, is more inclined to go after something not so much for themselves but more for those whom they protect.

They are the survivors of the world—the guys and gals who make a plan, who get things done. "My Way"[1] by Frank Sinatra, the well-known Eight singer, pretty much sums up an Eight's approach to life. They have this ability to protect the weak at their highest levels (think Schindler in the movie *Schindler's List*), but as they grow less healthy, they can also become bullies.

As they get more stressed, they can become increasingly bad-tempered. They can rage like a bull, only to have forgotten the incident (if they see themselves as having been victorious) moments afterwards. They don't like losing. Ever. If they feel they have been wronged they will appear to withdraw but, in reality, are waiting for the appropriate moment to exact revenge. Uplifting others slides into domineering others. They'll say things like: "When the going gets tough, the tough get going!" "Don't question me." "It's my way or the highway." Or the classic Al Capone quote, "Don't mistake my kindness for weakness. I'm kind to everyone, but when someone is unkind to me, weak is not what you're going to remember about me."

They start becoming extremely controlling and possessive over what they see as being theirs, including possessions and people. They become increasingly self-important and boost their achievements. They depersonalize others and can become intimidating and threatening to get what they want. As their feelings of vulnerability increase, they can wreak havoc in the lives of others in a megalomaniacal attempt to assert their dominance.

When they start acting out like unhealthy type Fives (isolating[2] and using anger to destroy others' ideas, beliefs, and so on), it's an indication that they are unhealthy. They become vengeful—outlaws who wish above anything to avenge those they believe have betrayed them. They won't care if they have upset a friend, waiter or family member; they want supreme control and start losing any humane feelings toward others.

Healthy Eights are courageous, resourceful, warm, generous, honorable, and forgiving, uplifting others with open, loving hearts.

Career Choices

You'll find them as site managers, truck drivers, bodyguards, middle managers, entrepreneurs (particularly if they have a Seven wing), salesmen and sales directors, politicians, marketing managers, department managers, army sergeants, property developers, boxers, warlords, restaurant owners, chefs, crime bosses (think Mafia bosses), even religious gurus. They won't enjoy loads of detail and paperwork and being the much-scrutinized office junior.

Eating Triggers

Type Eights have a lusty relationship with life. If they see something they desire, they want it immediately! They also have issues with survival. Put the two together, and you have someone who can go after what they want (and this includes food) with the passion that says, "My well-being depends upon it."

More = security and not feeling vulnerable, so it stands to reason then that Eights like to feel that there is always lots available and even if they lack the financial resources, they will beg, borrow, or steal to feel fulfilled and get what they want. As one Eight used to say to me, "I owe, I owe, so it's off to work I go!" Feeling that they want something but can't have it, as in "I want the 20-ounce rump steak but only can afford a burger," will see them inevitably ordering the steak, irrespective of the consequences. Feelings of vulnerability, not being in control, or trapped can trigger a desire to binge. It can also occur when they are super-angry, and they gorge mindlessly, as they plot and plan a counterattack.

How Eights Approach Eating

Eights are not fussy eaters, so fine dining with fiddly dishes makes little sense to them. Food must be as big and bold as they are. So the 72-ounce steak with extra french fries and a good bottle of red wine or a couple of beers would satisfy their lusty craving.

They are seldom concerned with health issues and don't feel guilty ordering the largest and best on the menu. Food is another way to dominate and be competitive with others, so if you order the 18-ounce sirloin steak, it's important to them to rule by choosing the 35-ounce option.

Just as they are lusty in life, so Eights are lusty in the way they eat. They will all too quickly forget the eating plan, when they see something on the menu or in the store that they desire.

Eights Eating Out

Eights can easily overindulge when they eat, as their passionate cravings rule. I've eaten out with an Eight who would order way more dishes than we could possibly eat (and yes, they will happily take it upon themselves to order for you), simply because they wanted a bit of whatever appealed. Whereas you or I might make a choice between what we thought sounded good, the Eight just ordered all appealing choices! Eights feel they deserve this indulgence—they have "brought home the bacon," so now they deserve to pig out as a reward.

Eights tend to push against the world. In a restaurant environment, this can translate into strolling into the kitchen and demanding food be served faster or confronting a waiter who they consider has slighted them in some way. Sometimes, it's difficult for others to see if the Eight is just being provocative in a humorous way or if they really mean business.

When I ate out with one Eight who was impatient about the table service, he called the restaurant's manager on his mobile. When the manager answered the phone, the Eight said: "Your service is bad. I need a waiter now at table seven." This is typical of an Eight. Naturally, the manager, followed by a trail of waiters, came scuttling to our table.

Knowing their own needs well, Eights make decisions fast, and you won't find them idly gazing at the menu trying to decide between the meat or the pasta. They know what they want and believe they also know what you want as well!

They are often the life and soul of the table—present and enjoying every minute of the occasion (but can be overbearing to some of the more sensitive types).

No-nonsense food or food that is not finicky will most likely be enjoyed by Eights. A quail egg with a dab of sauce and a lettuce leaf will be frustrating. They typically enjoy meat. They enjoy getting "bang for their buck," so may look for special treatment, discounts, or unique food preparation.

Eights Entertaining at Home

Type Eights who lean toward their Nine wings are particularly keen to be the king at the table surrounded by family or close friends, often in a more intimate environment;[3] whereas, Eights with a Seven wing will probably prefer hitting the city, clubbing, and "painting the town red" with a bunch of friends. They particulalry don't enjoy guests who accept an invitation and then don't arrive.

Eights enjoy get-togethers, where they can entertain their family and friends lavishly. Their sensuous natures carry over into food preparation, with its big and bold flavors. Gordon Ramsay, the famous TV chef, is I'm guessing, a good example of an Eight chef. Strong, willful, with a ferocious temper, he is not afraid to confront slackers and get things working his way. Be warned: Eights get really angry at guests who don't pitch up.

An Eight's home, like themselves, will be warm and inviting. If they have a Nine wing, they may be art lovers[4] and adorn their walls with bold, expressive, bright artworks (as opposed to sensitive etchings).

A simple barbeque at my Eight neighbor's house will see large filet and sirloin steaks, chicken kebabs, lamb chops, bacon/pork kebabs, and a table laden with salads of every variety. And this, after the starters. You're not going to leave an Eight's home hungry!

Food Choices

Because Eights are acquisitive, they generally love shopping, often with family or friends. An Eight I know lives in a country where foreign goods are hard to come by. Consequently, when out of his homeland, he spends most of his time in shopping malls. Days after he arrives at his holiday home here, trucks start arriving delivering a vast assortment of goods. Kitchen gadgets are a favorite purchase, along with an assortment of gourmet foods.

Eights enjoy the feeling that what they are buying is rare or exclusive; it creates added desirability. It excites them to feel they need to hunt harder to capture the product. If it's too easily available, and there's no victory in getting it, they can lose interest. Great food must be won to feel like a champion. If an Eight hears about a winery that only produces 50 bottles a year, the competition is on to get it. Limitation equals desirability.

Few Type Eights are vegetarians. In their world, where "eat or be eaten" is the rule, eating meat simply translates as winning the battle or the fittest having survived. They may be persuaded to stop eating meat for health reasons, but I've seldom found an Eight whose heart is really in the choice.

Remember that Lust is their Enneagram Passion. (Passion is used in the old context of the word in the Enneagrams. It is the behavior that causes our suffering, as in The Passion (pain) of Christ, which then becomes our ego fixation. Being caught up in our passion stops us from experiencing wholeness.) They relate to the biblical Seven Deadly Sins plus an additional two passions, deceit (Three) and fear/anxiety (Six).

In Type Eights, the Passion of Lust translates as going after what they want with immediacy. The Eight is the person who walks into a shop, looks around, assesses the options, chooses an item, and hauls out the credit card with no hesitation. They like the feeling of craving something and then getting it, so food desirability becomes a bit like desiring to have sex with someone (*I want it. I need it. How best to win it (fast)?*). At this point, cost is of little concern. Like foreplay, the sensuous desirability of the food becomes important. "These fresh oysters that just arrived this morning are stunning. We only have 40 left" are words sure to excite an Eight. Like sex, they want tantalizing, sensuous, juicy and flirtatious food.

What You May Not See

Eights hide their fear of being vulnerable under a thick armor of bravado. It's hard for others to believe sometimes that under this tough, confident, no-nonsense exterior lies a small archetypal child, longing for nurturance and intimacy. They don't want to appear needy in any way. When they feel someone "gets" them or "has their back," they can defend that person to the bitter end. A softer side of the Eight starts emerging, which can be both caring and loving. You're unlikely too to see guilt after a binge—Eights seldom feel it.

How Eights View Their Bodies

Most Eights are not too concerned about their appearance, although those with a Type Seven wing may be more dress-conscious or flashily dressed. Eights have a "take-it-or-leave-it" approach when it comes to dress.[5] When feeling good and in control, they will tend to dress with more style than when things are not going well for them. A bit like street fighters, less healthy Eights will not have an issue with wearing a torn T-shirt or jeans—in a sense, looking like they have just had a fight.

Because they are extremely confident, Eights will often view themselves as better looking than they are. Their confidence has them believing that they deserve wealth, power, and an attractive partner. They enjoy the feeling of being alpha males and females, stronger physically and shrewder mentally than those around them. In relation to their bodies, this can translate as going into a sport or adventurous situation others may steer clear of, or they may push themselves too hard, believing they are invincible, until a heart attack or stroke proves otherwise.

Eights often have rugged or rough features with a large build (think Donald Trump). Weakness is not on their radar, so they need their bodies to look imposing—to carry weight so they can throw their weight around (they may even wear large, chunky, bling jewellery to add to this overall feel).[6] A weak body means that they may need to be dependent on other people. This is not a comfortable feeling for an Eight, who seeks independence and self-reliance. Their body is the tool they use in the world to feel in control and to look imposing.

Eights can often ignore their physical ailments. "I'm too busy to go to the doctor," they yell at concerned partners. They may go for months with a pain and do nothing (being tough— "cowboys don't cry," and so forth).[7] Their lifestyle can make them prime candidates for heart disease.

Addictions

Eights are Type A personalities who push themselves hard, believing they are invincible.[8] Worrying little about the future and loving rich foods and alcohol in quantity can lead to addictions without the Eight really being aware of it. "I just party big" may disguise an addiction. They can also have the belief that "I'm bigger than whatever substance it is others believe I'm addicted to." As a result, they may believe they don't need help—*I'm strong. I can handle this, or stop whenever I want to* type of thinking—and avoid getting help. It is extremely hard for them to admit they are not in control of their addictive desires. Getting help equates to not being able to handle the situation, which as you've come to understand is not desirable.

If they do embark on a recovery program, it will be on their terms. They will try to control the group and intimidate facilitators, as well as be outright confrontational with those they see stepping out of line. In an unhealthy state, they can create cronyism and cliques to undermine the power of those who seek to help them.[9]

They need to understand that confrontation and honesty (calling a spade a spade) alone is not sufficient, but needs to be accompanied by love in order to demonstrate true power. When they allow themselves to be humble, vulnerable, and genuinely seek support, they are well on the path to recovery.

Childhood

What we repress as children, because we felt it was somehow not acceptable, becomes our shadow self, which we then project onto the outside world. So it is that the strong, invincible Eight feels that they are surrounded by weak, needy others.[10] Eights had to repress this vulnerable aspect of themselves as children. "Boys don't cry" was the type of message they received, often from parents who themselves were fighting their own addictive battles.

They may have suffered abuse as children, or watched others they cared about being abused, making them determined to be strong and never have to experience the same pain they felt being victims. They may have found themselves having to care for younger siblings, assuming the leadership and protector role not provided by parents. Having to be in charge meant often denying their own needs, even to the extent of undergoing extreme hardships with little complaint. If life was particularly hard and they received little nurturance, they can become ferociously independent as adults, determined not to rely on anyone or anything.

Foodwise, this translates into being determined not to need anything from anyone—a Bear Grylls approach to life, where they can be totally self-reliant yet with others reliant on them. Like this popular TV program, Man vs Wild (previously called Born Survivor) survival issues are what motivate the Eight—what doesn't kill you makes you stronger.

Diets for Eights

Food is the fuel that strengthens Eights to do battle. It's the way they can "carry weight." When an Eight walks into the consulting rooms of a dietitian or a doctor, they will be in full-on defense mode. Being in this situation will make them feel vulnerable, and as we know, Eights loathe feelings of weakness and vulnerability.

They may view someone who wants them to lose weight as wanting them to lose power. As a result, Eights can be intimidating, especially to types who shy away from confrontation, or who have not worked with Eights before.[11] Left to their own devices, they'll soon have the practitioner dancing to their tune. This will understandably not serve them. To counter this attack, a practitioner will need to verbalize in a nonaggressive way but nevertheless shooting from the hip, that they sense the Eight's anger and suggest that their intensity would be better focused on their health issues.

They enjoy laying down the law, but don't enjoy the reverse. They need to feel in control, and that includes what they eat. If they themselves decide to forego steak, that's fine; tell them that they can't eat it and you're waving a red flag at a bull. Get their buy-in, and you've got a better chance of success. Self-restraint is not a word usually associated with Eights.

As noted earlier, Eights have a lust for life. What they desire they want (and they want it now!). This thinking is not conducive to the restrictions imposed by diets. The Eight will be after instant gratification and immediate results ("I haven't eaten carbs for a week, and I'm only down half a pound. This program isn't working"). For them, inspiration will come from understanding that by optimizing their health, they will be less vulnerable. Being healthy means being stronger and sexier, two things Eights aspire to be. A person at peak fitness can stand up to others with greater conviction than someone who is weaker. If they understand this, then they will buy into the program, with the strength, intensity, and conviction that is part of their nature.

Exercise

"Survival of the fittest" is their motto. To be fitter, though, involves dedication. Eights are happy to do this if they see the rewards in terms of being made captain, winning matches, and gaining in strength and power. They love to lead, so will work hard to achieve this in the team. Sports involving physical contact, such as rugby, karate, judo, kick boxing, water polo, ice hockey, wrestling, or boxing will be popular. They enjoy the intensity and feelings of aliveness that comes with combat sports. Although it does not have the satisfaction of hand-to-hand combat, weightlifting involves gaining mass and muscle, which Eights enjoy. It also affirms their body as being a shield against worldly threats and makes them feel more invincible.

Winning against the odds is hugely satisfying for Eights; it confirms their strength and power, the victim made hero. Eights with a Seven wing will be drawn to more adventurous sports, such as big wave surfing, base jumping, parachuting, powerboat racing, motorbike racing, and kitesurfing. Merely partaking in these sports gives them street credibility.

They are more likely to stick to an exercise program if defeating others is at its core rather than simply doing it for themselves. Eights are very competitive. Emotional intensity translates into physical intensity, which Eights enjoy. At its best, this need to dominate can drive a team to higher levels of achievement. At its worst, it becomes bullying and blaming of the weaker members with recriminations and sulking and even deferred frustrated anger, such as lashing out at someone who may have had nothing to do with the actual sporting event. A feeling of lack of success in life can drive them to try even harder to achieve on the sportsfield.

There may be clashes with coaches or team captains if the Eight feels the coach or captain is limiting or restricting their performance in any way, or simply because they believe they would make a stronger leader. Being told to do something a certain way will seldom work for an Eight (they'd rather that job be left to them!). They can then undermine those in leadership roles.

Should they lose, particularly in a one-to-one sport, Eights may well withdraw to stew and, against their normally "out there" nature, silently plan a revenge match. You may have won the battle, but they'll be planning to win the war! Seeking justice quickly turns to needing to revenge a loss. In this instance, they may decide to train alone, rather than with a group, in order to hide their vulnerability while they shrewdly devise a game plan and master any new techniques.

How to Inspire Eights

You may find Eights are initially unwilling participants in a weight-loss program. They don't want to feel vulnerable and not in charge, so they may attempt to undermine your position by covert or openly angry behavior. If you can understand the situation for what it is and not be intimidated, you can inspire them through understanding that being fitter and stronger, they can experience a greater sense of authentic power and feel more able to protect themselves.[12]

Impress upon them that true power comes with helping the downtrodden rather than stamping on them. Translation: true heroes are only heroes because they are courageous, forgiving, loving, and selfless.

Levels of Health

Healthy

When Eights are at their best, they can turn even the most adverse situations into opportunities to grow and reinvent themselves. This includes health issues. They are self-motivated to make the best of themselves, so will stick with an eating plan, workout, and do whatever else it takes to remain physically and emotionally healthy. Healthy Eights may turn to uplifting others whom they feel may have suffered as they have done. They could be the inspirational but kindly coach helping disadvantaged kids or championing the cause of the underdog. Here their magnanimous heart shines brightly. True heroes, they no longer feel the need to control their world. They can rein in their appetites, give up their need to be the captain of the team, and are happy to serve others.

Average

As Eights become less healthy, life appears as more of a challenge to be met with streetwise toughness; it becomes "me against the world." Exercise becomes about toughening up rather than just a desire to be fit. Eating is about taking on board the fuel for the fight. Big is better, and that goes for portion sizes and biceps. The need to control others increases.

Eights, like Type Twos, may binge, using food to stuff their feelings down (in their case, feelings of vulnerability). They start to mask their true feelings, such as pretending to the opposition that their team's loss means nothing when, in fact, it means everything. They start boosting themselves by puffing themselves up, regaling others with tales of victories and potential winning strategies. Now, as they head into battle, they look behind them to see if they are being supported and may berate others for not doing so. Their tendency toward anger increases and erupts in violent outbursts, even to the point of being threatening and demanding compliance.

Unhealthy

Lust for whatever they desire at whatever cost dominates over reason and reasonableness. They can become destructive toward others, but equally, direct that approach inward, toward themselves. Eating badly, eating too much of the wrong food, and drinking bouts where no limits are the rule can seriously jeopardize their health (and don't even consider telling them to stop). Anger explodes in road rage, picking fights, and deliberately wanting to harm opposing team players in dirty play. If you beat them, beware of the next encounter. Heart and blood-pressure issues can arise, as they drive themselves relentlessly and become dangerous and defiant. That big, warm heart has become hard.

If Eights are able to recognize when they are unhealthy, they can accept the child within who feels that they have to defend themselves against the world. It's no longer me *against* them; it's me *with* them. They experience the true power that only comes from love. Thus, they rise from power-mongering warlords to become courageous heroes—on the field, in the office, and in confronting their own demons: innocent and pure, merciful and magnanimous.

Summary

Lusty Eights need to understand that following a healthier lifestyle will reward them with feeling stronger and even more capable and confident. Focusing on better not bigger portions will help. Understanding that they are doing this for themselves, rather than to please others, will lessen resistance.

If you make a healthier lifestyle a challenge you want to win rather than something that limits your experience in the world, it will go a long way to helping you achieve your goal. Make competition a pastime. You'll be inspired to push yourself harder if the reward of victory is at stake. Use your success to inspire and uplift others who may not have the same commitment and drive that you have.

Certain health insurance companies, as noted earlier, now have online forums where you can compete with others and feel supported by them, and in turn, be supportive in your individual goals. Make the changes needed to allow yourself to feel more alive and, when you resist temptation, stronger. Experiment with salads rather than steak. Use your inner resourcefulness to discover a healthier you. Healthier = true survival ability!

Type Nine
Sluggish Scoffer or the Serene Health-Seeker

The Issue

Type Nines unconsciously stuff down their anger with food. Wanting to keep the peace necessitates suppressing their anger. Not wanting to acknowledge or feel anger translates as a numbing to self, resulting in disengagement and disconnection from the physical body. Being disconnected from their physical selves, they tend to eat fast and finish the plate, even if they were actually full when they were only halfway through it. Some Nines can be very overweight (from eating unconsciously), while others can be painfully skinny (from ignoring the body's hunger needs and forgetting to eat).

Overview of Type Nine

Type Nines are relaxed, likeable, and easy-going. They feel unthreatening and as the name given to them in the Riso/Hudson tradition of Peacemaker suggests, enjoy creating a harmonious atmosphere wherever they are. They are solid citizens, patient and steady, with an "I'll be there for you attitude."

They are uncomplicated, comforting, genial, and happy to blend into the surroundings, often having a serene and calm presence. They are afraid of being "tall poppies"—tall poppy syndrome or standing above others—and can impede their potential through an unconscious desire to remain small and therefore, not in a vulnerable top-dog position. This makes them humble to a fault. They are open, natural, and spontaneous, with an almost childlike playfulness when healthy.

To maintain the peace they desire, they often sublimate their own desires and anger and merge into the personalities of those around them. With a group of Type Fives, a Type Nine woman may be silent and studious but may become the "belle of the ball" at a party with Type Sevens. "I worked in advertising, home to many Sevens. It's easy to see why I thought I was one, given how I merged into the partying, fun lifestyle," recalls a Type Nine. They can sometimes be hard to identify, as a result of their ability to over-accommodate others, they appear to be a bit of many types.

Nines are homebodies who enjoy the comfort of a familiar couch and a loving pet. They have a calming and healing presence, which draws others to them. They make great steady and supportive friends, and while having difficulties voicing their own opinions, they can be assertive when it comes to their children, colleagues, or others close to them.

They are most often completely unaware of their suppressed anger. One Type Nine told me: "I went to this old German therapist who had me doing all sorts of tests. At the end, she gave me feedback saying that I had all this anger bottled up inside of me. I was confused. It didn't feel like that at all. It took 30 odd years before I realized that she had been right."

Although their Enneagram Passion is Laziness (Sloth[1]), this is often a laziness to show up for themselves rather than physical laziness (although it can be)—I've known marathon runners who are Nines. Nines are the low reactors of the world. Because of this, they often undergo a fair amount of emotional abuse, tension, and neglect, often from partners or office superiors who take them for granted, using them as emotional dumping grounds. Nines tend to go to sleep in an unhappy relationship rather than leave it.

For Nines, the glass is always half full—whether it's looking for parking or starting a new project, they expect things to work out. When they are healthier they work to make things happen the way they planned, but as they become less healthy, it becomes more hoping for the best. They'll enjoy pastimes such as vegetable gardening, art, reading, or watching a lot of TV.

Because they battle to express their anger (it implodes and only occasionally explodes), as they become less healthy, they can become passive-aggressive and stubborn. They don't want anything or anyone to shake their happy world. The desire to not face anything upsetting can make them emotionally unavailable—a sort of numbing out of reality.

Unhealthy Nines become downtrodden, helpless denialists, day-dreaming of a life they'll make little effort to make a reality. Resigned to their perceived fate, they'll stubbornly refuse all offers of help. They avoid problems, either by convincing themselves that they are above the issues of this earthly plane (false enlightenment) or huge denial (scaling down the importance of any negativity), walking through life in an ever more blinkered fashion and refusing to change.

Whereas we may have disintegrated blindly, with this information, integration is a choice.

Career Choices

Nines are often creative and imaginative. Their adaptability can see them in many different fields, and they may be involved in art, change to writing, get into sales, then become manufacturers. They generally don't enjoy working in corporations because of the office politics and so more frequently end up working for themselves. This is also because they loathe stress, so working from home with the dog at their feet and coffee on the boil suits their personality. If they lean more toward a Type Eight wing, they can make excellent leaders. They negotiate well, push from behind rather than needing (or wanting) to walk in front, yet the Eight's strength is there when needed.

They are steady workers who can throw themselves into work to avoid uncomfortable feelings. They avoid positions where there is potential conflict. As noted, you'll often find them working from home, or working as botanists, game wardens or park rangers (the outdoors is peaceful), veterinarians, writers, artists, musicians, teachers, yoga instructors, counselors, mediators, social workers, editors, and laid-back surfers. They can also make good alternative practitioners, as when healthy their simple presence can be healing.

Eating Triggers

Nines suppress their unhappiness, anxiety, turmoil, and anger because they don't want to create disharmony. As they numb out, mindlessly eat food, drink alcohol, and sometimes take drugs, this becomes the elixir to create peace and strengthen the bars around their inner sanctum. In this daydream space, they can eat and drink way too much without even realizing they are doing so. When stressed, they may completely deny having any health issues ("No I haven't been for my check-up; I've just been too busy." "I'm not obese; I'm just carrying a few extra pounds"). As with unhealthy Fives, they can neglect themselves, allowing others to exploit them.

To avoid feeling emotional pain, Nines numb themselves to what is happening around them, which can cause huge frustration for others who are demanding that they pay attention. They can typify the "elephant in the room" scenario ("Problem? What problem?"). Unable to act or express how they feel, food becomes a way for them to stuff down their anger.

How Nines Approach Eating

Type Twos use food to stuff down feelings of being unloved, whereas Nines use food to stuff down feelings of anger. It's easier to "eat one's anger" than express the rage. Hunger is never satisfied, because it's not a real hunger for food ("If there's food I eat it, but allow myself to be carried along with others' choices, not really taking any responsibility for what I eat"). Nines aren't too concerned about bad food choices. The long-term ramifications of a lifetime of bad eating somehow seem a far-off thing, and they are numbed in a fog of indifference.

They may have told themselves to avoid certain foods, but if everyone else is ordering pudding or cheesy pizza, those disciplines disappear sooner than you can say, "The one with extra cream is mine!" They tend to eat more than others—only when the plate is empty will they stop; they just aren't aware that they are full.

They are not too concerned with what they eat when alone. Less effort, more ease is the way to go, and that can mean takeout or raiding the fridge for whatever might be there. McDonald's Happy Meals were made for Nines!

Nines Eating Out

When it comes to getting ready to go out, Nines will inevitably get their priorities wrong and be doing something arbitrary rather than what is required to get ready. This habit means they are invariably late, which doesn't seem to concern them too much, unless, of course, their hosts display visible anger.

This was how a Nine described her timekeeping problem to me.

> "It's not that I plan to be late, but I just get involved with
> something else. Take going to art class, when the teacher
> asked us not to be late. Just before I'm about to leave
> I pop over to my neighbor to drop off something of hers.
> She asks me in for coffee, and I do a quick calculation and
> think I can just squeeze it in (I don't want to offend her).
> Then I'm just walking to my car when another neighbor
> stops for a chat. Before I know it, I'm going inside her
> home for a glass of wine, even though I know I now will be
> late for class. Eventually, I arrive 30 minutes late."

Nines who have strong One wings may be the exception, arriving on time to avoid upsetting their host (Ones don't like bad timekeeping).

At a cocktail party, because they eat unconsciously, Nines may only be slightly aware of the potato chips they are snacking on, and unaware that they are full, simply continue to eat what is in front of them. If the Nine is feeling alone or awkward, mindlessly snacking becomes a way of dealing with the discomfort.

When it comes to choosing a restaurant, even if they have a preference, Nines will be easily swayed ("Oh, you want curry? Okay, no problem. Let's go there then, rather than the pizza place"). Because in childhood they grew to believe that other people's needs were more important than their own, they will quickly back down, although perhaps slightly less so with Nines, who lean more toward Type Eight than Type One. Likewise, when it comes to table choice and so on, more Eightish Nines may take more of a lead in deciding where to sit, but most often, they'll leave the choice to someone else.

Nines will order what the group is having. They may not be sure what it is they really want or simply want to feel part of the group. You won't have them ordering the most expensive dish, even if they want to, because that would make them stand out. They will usually see what everyone else is ordering and go along with that, meaning that they are often one of the last people to order at the table.

But if they repeatedly end up eating sushi when they wanted steak, after many such experiences they may explode in rage—a rage their partner never saw coming. It's good for others in relationships with Nines to realize that they may have become so used to having their will imposed, they are not even aware that it's happening, or they may see their Nine partner as not minding at all where they go.

If the order for them arrives and is incorrect, they will most likely not bring attention to it and eat what they have been given. Disliking confrontation, they are mortified when others complain in restaurants.

Nines Entertaining at Home

The home of a Nine tends to be comfortable but cluttered. Like Type Fives, they can be hoarders (but for a different reason)—old magazines, potentially useful bits and bobs, broken watering cans, and so on. They hate throwing away what they may need one day. If living with a stronger partner, the home will more likely reflect their partner's style than their own. Animals happily sunning themselves on a sofa covered with the dog's hair would be typical, together with a worn but much-loved rug.

For Type Ones, in particular, this clutter and chaos can be unsettling. It's not that Nines don't clean; they do, but they get bored during the process and may not complete the job, or they may tidy a cupboard only to have it in a jumble within days.

Said one Nine: "Cleaning my home office is my worst task. I'll procrastinate any way possible to avoid doing it, yet when I do it feels great. By the close of play the following day, though, it's back to its old, cluttered state, so it seems rather pointless."

Some Nines really enjoy cooking, and take great care, as Twos would, to make sure each person's tastes are catered for; but as with all things, they seldom take the same care and attention when it comes to cooking for themselves and their needs.

They are gracious hosts and make guests feel relaxed, which is a wonderful gift that Nines have. Provided you don't mind a cat curled up on your lap or a drooling dog eyeing your lamb chop, you'll feel welcome and at home. Wanting to please, their food will be plentiful and unpretentious. If you are eating with a Nine who enjoys cooking, you'll enjoy a sensual balance of color and flavor. Don't be surprised if, at the end of the evening, they whip out a board or card game; many Nines love to play parlor games!

Food Choices

Weighed down by the choices of others, Nines seldom indulge their own food desires openly. However, if away from others, a Nine may rebel against this conformism and indulge in what they have wanted but not allowed themselves to have. "I enjoyed going by the stationery store to buy supplies for the office," a Nine recalls, "because there was a restaurant next door where I could order caramel cheesecake and a large cappuccino without feeling I was being judged by others. It became a sort of fun adventure I would never have had under the critical eye of my partner or colleagues."

Away from family and friends, their stifled individuality emerges and appears as the curry the family generally finds too hot, the burger their health-conscious wife would disapprove of, or the forbidden slab of chocolate that makes them happy. Because Nines are generally such nice people, others often have no idea of the extent to which the Nine has sublimated their tastes and choices to keep everyone happy.

If Nines opt for being vegetarian or vegan, it's often because it is the path of least resistance if their partner or group of friends have strong opinions on the matter, or simply a way to make for a happier world ("Eating meat, after I've seen the videos of the poor animals, makes me uncomfortable, so I'd rather not").

Doing the household shopping can be a lengthy affair, as Nines ponder both the economics of one product over another, versus what the family would most like to eat ("John likes mixed frozen vegetables, but Jen will only eat peas. What to do?").

What You May Not See

What many people don't see is that Nines are very independent people. They like doing their own thing in their own happy worlds; consequently, they don't enjoy clingy or needy partners. Constantly subverting their needs and desires to fit in with those of others builds up a huge pile of anger, and this causes a dilemma, because to voice their frustration means to disturb the peace, which they don't want to do.

"We never fight," a Nine told me proudly, regarding his marriage. When I suggested that this was not necessarily healthy, he was horrified. He could not see the extent to which he was angry.

What people often don't understand, though, is that appearing to have no or few needs doesn't stop Nines from wanting their needs met. If a partner or friend does not understand this, rather than make a demand, a Nine will withdraw into their own "happy" world and may well attempt to suppress their unhappiness with eating and drinking. Others will then just experience them as remote or removed, without getting what the problem is. Nines themselves often don't understand the connection.

Behind the pleasing, happy, and relaxed façade, there is (in less emotionally healthy Nines) a huge dragon waiting to breathe fire. Recognizing this and working with it can reconnect heart, mind, and body and in releasing the anger, the need to stuff it down with food and addictions.

Type Nines enjoy food, especially if they have the wing of an earthy, lusty Type Eight. But because they are not aware of their bodies, they may unconsciously undereat or overeat.

How They View Their Bodies

Not wanting to address uncomfortable issues, Nines who are not happy with their bodies will simply avoid looking in the mirror ("New Age blurb kept on telling me to stand in front of a full-length mirror and 'love my body.' I didn't feel that I loved my body any more by staring at it. Rather, I got along much better with it if I ignored its lumps and bumps").

Seeing rolls of fat would disturb their happy space, so Nines simply gloss over it. There is a feeling of resignation about the way they look, as if their fate is to be overweight, and that's just how it is.

Their main source of discomfort would be being so fat that they feel too different from their friends or colleagues. They want to blend in, and being fat won't allow this ("I was very unhappy with my weight. I thought about it constantly, but never seemed to feel powerful enough to actually tackle the problem").

Being positive in their outlook, Nines can override their feelings of sadness at their appearance with a cheery "Fat people are happier" or as a Nine school matron told me: "When I was young I thought I was fat but wasn't really. Now I am really fat and long to be fat like I thought I was back then."

Nines can sometimes see their bodies as pieces of meat, rather than as divine temples. Being in their bodies (or in touch with them) can connect with their anger, which they want to avoid. They want to be comfortable; anger is uncomfortable. It's easier then to be numb to their body and its needs. Habits and routines become a way of going to sleep.

Nines are neglectful of themselves, and this can take a bizarre turn. For instance, I've heard some Nines say that they avoid going to the bathroom if they are involved with something, even though they may want to urinate badly. Likewise, they may want a drink of water but not get themselves one, or if they are in physical pain, be able to switch it off. Such is a Nine's lack of self-focus.

"I broke my leg in two places. When I tried to stand up, it was so sore, without thinking, I swore like mad. It was very painful. Yet once I managed to get a lift home, my husband thought it was just a twisted ankle. When we got to the hospital, they marked me as a code green, which in my hospital triage or SATS system means, on a scale 1 to 10 of emergency, it's 0–2 i.e. nothing much wrong here, wasting hospital time. The doctor said it was a sprain but eventually agreed with an x-ray (I didn't yell when he twisted my ankle, even though it was excruciating).

Kids with coughs, stitch removals—everyone was seen before I was. It was only when I wanted to go to the loo and they told me to walk there, which was impossible, that they took some notice. This was in a private hospital. Eventually, almost 4 hours after my admission, I was taken to be x-rayed. Suddenly, after seeing the extent of the two breaks, the staff sprang into action and I was wheeled into a ward to await surgery and given morphine. Next time, I'll yell a bit. I've learnt grinning and bearing it doesn't work!"

Nines are often sensual people, but they don't want their sensuousness to draw attention to themselves; whereas some other numbers would enjoy the attention, Nines would feel awkward about it. In relationships, they want to avoid the pain of rejection, so may cut off from another person rather than risk rejection, like a Three. The sensuality is often expressed, though, in the way they eat and cook (think of Nigella Lawson, the TV chef).

Addictions

Booze is a great way to water down anger, while dope[2] creates the chilled space that a Nine seeks. Alcoholics typically enjoy their addiction because, after a couple of drinks, the world becomes a happier, friendlier place. The stranger sitting next to you at the bar becomes your mate, you feel the pain of failure less, and literally see the world through rosé-tinted glasses, just as Nines love to do! It also encourages you to come out of your shell and be more gregarious and friendly. But it can also lead to a Nine vegging out in front of the TV, paying no attention to their real needs, as they down another beer and munch a slice of pizza. Or they head to the pub and repeat the same stories to the same bunch of mates in an alcohol-induced, spaced-out zone.

As they disintegrate, Nines become more ineffectual and eventually, in the worst cases, catatonic. They want to avoid acknowledging that everything is not alright with them. Drugs become a way to avoid confronting problems such as anxiety, repressed anger, being alone, or the frustration and anger of others directed toward them.

In rehabilitation, a Nine will appear to be the model addict, agreeing with all the rules and suggestions. They don't enjoy any form of conflict and should it occur, they will zone out into their own happy, anesthetized world. If the outside world becomes too threatening for them to remain in their daydream world, they may revert to their addiction.

Childhood

Nines often report having childhoods where they were largely ignored, possibly because of a younger sibling or their parents' preoccupation with another interest. They learn to fly under the radar so as not to become the target for any anger that may be flying around the home. They often experienced fighting parents, so becoming inconspicuous became a way to survive. The little Nine learnt that to be safe you didn't take sides, but rather numbed out and let the conflict rage around you. Yet, ask a Nine about their childhood and most of the time, as in other aspects of their lives, they'll describe it as being happy. It's often only in therapy that a different picture emerges.

"My parents bickered endlessly," said a Nine. "It was always about such petty issues. They were both control freaks and had to prove that their opinion was correct. As a result, even in my teenage years, I took refuge in my tree-hut with a book and my cat."

Another gave this description of her childhood: "My mother wanted me to take her side against my father. I would do so when with her, but then would feel disloyal when with him. I literally felt pulled apart, yet I didn't have the courage to stand up to them both and tell them to sort it out and not involve me. Being friendly to both of them became the best way for me to keep the peace and not run the threat of having one or other get angry with me. I never considered that I might have an actual opinion."

A Type Nine told us in a workshop about how, as a child of seven returning from holiday, he had broken his leg exploring a cave. His parents did not want to be inconvenienced by having to stop at that town's hospital and decided instead to drive the children the five hours back to their home town. The man described how he had sat in the car in excruciating pain, not wanting to complain, which would have angered his parents.

Another Nine described going on a picnic with his three siblings when he was four. The family forgot all about him, and it was only when they were home that they realized that they had left him behind. These are typical stories of a Type Nine childhood.

Just as they are often overlooked in the family, so too are their needs. They may want the chicken, but will happily eat the eggs given to them, if that's what's going to make Mom happy. This goes for finishing their food, even if they are full. It's better than running the risk of being accused of not being appreciative.

Diets for Nines

Nines enjoy comfort rather than change. They don't like it if life becomes too difficult or disrupted; they prefer a chilled relax-on-the-couch-with-the-cat lifestyle. So tell a Nine that they need to change their comfortable routine by eating differently and adding exercise to the equation and you're not going to get too much enthusiasm, other than what they need to show so as not to upset you. They may zone out into their happy space by telling long stories that while away their appointment time but don't allow for any real confrontation of the problem.

Because much of a Nine's eating happens in a zoned-out space, they can eat when full and eat too fast so that their appestat doesn't have a chance to kick in. They go with the flow, so if everyone else is eating or drinking a particular way, Nines will happily drop their agreed-on diet and do as everyone else is doing. Even if the Nine wants to stick to a diet, if everyone at the office is having Friday drinks, it normally doesn't take much to twist the arm of an affable Nine, to have them ordering a gin and tonic with the rest of the gang. Likewise, at home, if their partner likes to eat in a certain way, Nines mostly will follow suit, even if they don't particularly enjoy the food.

For example, in one instance, a Nine's partner started eating only steak and the same salad for both lunch and supper. This Nine loved cooking and was good at it. At first she resisted but got tired of making her own meals, so she soon fell into the eating pattern of her partner, even though she did not like steak or salad prepared that way. It was easier just to go along with things.

The path of least resistance becomes the Nine's way of eating. They don't value their bodies or themselves enough to speak out for what will be the healthier option. They may also find it a drag to have to weigh portions or prepare anything special for themselves (even if they do this for others). When everyone else's needs are more important than your own, you'd sooner cook for the family than make a low-fat meal for yourself. As a result, they will eat leftovers or whatever is to hand. They'll cook a great meal to please family or friends, but left to their own devices to eat for themselves, the stew from a few days ago will be just fine!

Another way a Nine's zoned-out approach to food and dieting can manifest is that they may start out with all guns blazing and on a mission to change, but get waylaid. For example, they may start to make a batch of healthy muesli for breakfast but get lost somewhere in the process between buying the ingredients and actually completing the task. Or they may understand that they have a problem with being overweight, but not really acknowledge that lack of exercise or diet plays a large factor in this and needs to be addressed.

Some offices have sweet jars that get regularly replenished. This is bad news for the nice Nine who will unconsciously grab a couple on the way past. They are particularly susceptible to sweeter food, as if in choosing sweets, they long for life to be sweeter.

When working with Nines, dietitians and doctors must realize that they need to make food choices simple—for example, a breakfast smoothie made with a few simple ingredients would work. As I've mentioned, Nines often resist changes, and this includes the way they eat. But if they do get used to a new way of eating, then they can stick to it because change again would disrupt their happy space.

Nines may start a diet full of good intentions, but when the results aren't instant, many quickly slip back into their old habits, giving up and feeling that there is no hope in continuing.

Said one Nine: "Every New Year, I'd tell myself that I would lose weight; every year, I'd end up putting on more. I battled with commitment, and attempts seldom lasted longer than a couple of weeks. I gave up on myself. It was easier to just accept my fat body than do something about it. That was until my partner started eating healthily. I resisted joining him for at least 10 months, before I thought, *What the heck!* and joined him. That was a turning point for me."

Nines can be extremely stubborn in a passive aggressive show of rebelliousness. As a result they may 'delay' starting a diet or simply refuse to be goaded into one.

The appestat is a hypothetical region of the brain, most likely located in the hypothalamus or near the pituitary gland. Its function is to help regulate the appetite. If you are aware of your body, which most Nines are not, you will listen to your body's feeling of being full and stop eating. When functioning optimally, this appestat, together with the adipostat[3] (believed to be a series of hormonal outputs), tells the brain that you're full. However, the message can be easily overridden, particularly when you eat too quickly. By eating too fast you've finished a whole lot more food than you need before this message can come into play. Even if you do eat fast, eat less, and although you initially may still feel hungry after a meal, when your appestat does kick in, you'll feel full. If you feel full before

20 minutes have passed, it's a sure indication that you've bitten off way more food than you need to chew. Its interesting that in not absorbing and digesting food adequately Nines mirror not absorbing or digesting uncomfortable feelings.

Nines are also great procrastinators if they aren't healthy. So they may ponder a diet but find excuses to delay getting started ("I'll wait until after my birthday." "I'm busy with work now, so when I'm not so busy I'll start"). Years can pass with no action being taken. It helps hugely then for a Nine to have a "hands on," motivating person close at hand.

"For me," said a Nine, "the dietitian's focus on losing centimeters rather than kilograms was a huge shift. No more scale watching and the resultant guilt afterwards. I stuck to the eating program (no weighed food, either, which was great) and exercised twice a week, and the centimeters melted away. Keep it simple, so it's easy to follow."

Nines fall easily into routines, so setting up a program with a simple routine, after a couple of weeks becomes easy for them to follow.

Exercise

As a rule, you're more likely to find Nines in front of the computer, watching TV, or playing board games than on the sportsfield or at the gym. They typically are more sedentary than the other types, not competitive (unless they have moved to their Type Three aspect), and battle with organizing their time to fit in playing regular sport. As they become less healthy emotionally, they lose passion for life and can't seem to drum up the motivation to be active. Persistence in things they don't enjoy is also not one of their strengths, so good intentions can easily fall by the wayside.

Some Nines engage in sport or activities to avoid uncomfortable feelings. Being busy playing sports or leaving a toxic home environment to take a long-distance run are very good ways of conflict avoidance. It's acceptable to engage in these activities, so a significant other can't really get angry with them for taking time out for training, even if the partner may suspect it's a means of avoidance.

Those Nines who are not couch potatoes tend to enjoy long-lasting, slow-burn sports rather than those that involve sudden bursts of speed or action. So long-distance running will take preference over sprinting. Gardening is a popular pastime and great to encourage activity and getting outdoors. Most Nines have green fingers and a natural affinity for plants and nature.

Nines often enjoy exercise more if they do it with others. If a few friends are doing yoga classes, Nines could well join too, because it feels like a fun, social thing to do. They delight even more in having coffee with the group afterwards—the inclination is more about being with someone else than achieving the actual weight goal particularly for Social Nines.

"I started walking 8km a day because it was a good way to spend time with a close friend who was far more fitness conscious than myself. I really look forward to the time away from my desk, the chats we have, and in particular, the coffee afterwards. Without her, I know I would have slacked off and found 101 reasons not to exercise."

If a group of friends or colleagues is not available, then a personal trainer with whom the Nine has a good connection can work as well. This other person(s) can play an important role on the road to fitness. If they are aware of this, Nines can use the information to motivate them to join a club, class, or get together with a committed friend(s) who have a similar fitness level. Even if they may dread the actual training session, they feel very chuffed about having attended.

As I noted earlier, my health insurance company in South Africa is aware of this buddy system and has made it possible to have online buddies to compare and encourage each other to reach goals. Some large companies offer wellness incentive plans for their employees. It would be wonderful if more companies took heed of the importance of this process, particularly for their Nine members.

As their Enneagram Passion of Sloth or Laziness suggests, Nines are not naturally inclined to be active, unless they find a sport they really enjoy, which will most likely not be at the gym. They may tell themselves to take a walk, but their habit of watching a favorite TV show will in most cases win out. Nines enjoy routines, so if they get into a regular exercise date, with the added input of a group of people they enjoy being with, they can stick to it. External forces can be motivators, such as wanting to lose weight to attract a certain partner, or having to reach a certain level of fitness to enter the police force.

High intensity training (HIT) workouts are not for them. They will be more attracted to slower-paced types of exercise, such as yoga (many end up as yoga teachers), tai chi, surfing, or even swimming at their own pace.

Both Nines with a One wing and Nines with an Eight wing may struggle to stay focused on their weight goals. While Nines with a One wing can be energetic, they can easily get side-tracked. For example: "I was going to the gym, but then the phone rang, and once I'd dealt with that, then I realized I had to stop off at the shops for supper, so I never made it to exercise." Nines with Eight wings are more inclined to enjoy comfort, so the couch may take preference over the gym. They often have a sort of slow, lumbering walk and can have slightly hooded or sleepy eyes like Dean Martin. They are more likely to be overweight, whereas Nines with One wings are more likely to be too thin.

If a Nine can see that their sedentary lifestyle will have long-term consequences, they can be persuaded to change rather than face the discomfort of bad health.

As one Nine explained: "When the dietitian clearly showed me, based on my blood tests, that I was very close to having Type 2 diabetes, and told me the consequences of having it, I realized I had to do something about my weight and general health. I had reached the tipping point. I could not avoid the issue any longer. I often dread my exercise routine, but know I have to stick to it."

Nines may bumble along, not really pushing themselves to be better. If they're okay enough to be in the team, they're happy. If they are in a team (and they make good team players), they will not want to upset the team by performing badly, neither will they want to outshine their teammates and draw too much attention to themselves. The desire not to let the team down, though, is in itself a good motivator; they may even stop themselves from winning (often unconsciously sabotaging themselves), so as not to upset others.

One good suggestion to help Nines bring greater awareness to exercise is to get one of these watches that beeps every hour if you have not done 200 steps 10 000 steps a day. A Type Five would ignore the beep in favor of the project they were working on, but a Nine could be encouraged to follow the beep to weight loss and fitness.

Levels of Health

Healthy

Emotionally healthy Nines are unselfconscious, imaginative, dynamic, life-embracing, humble, natural, relaxed, imaginative, and serene. This translates into being aware and present. They no longer snack mindlessly, but eat according to what their bodies require. They are physically and emotionally self-aware and no longer hide behind a pleasant pastime.

Being able to act, they no longer procrastinate when it comes to taking up a fitness routine or eating more healthily and are receptive to input from professionals. Gone are the dreamy expectations; instead, they are able to energetically create attainable goals. They are aware of when their anger arises and able to voice their opinion (in the nicest way!).

Average

As they become less healthy, Nines start losing passion for life, and with it the inclination to alter their comfortable routines in any way. If they have always run, then they can happily continue to do so, but it may take a lot to get them motivated to start something new.

People-pleasing starts to replace authenticity. Disengaging from themselves in order to fit in with others, Nines start to repress anything that may upset the status quo and (unconsciously) look for ways to suppress anger. They procrastinate about starting a weight-loss program and stop making exercise a priority. They may begin making excuses to avoid meeting up with friends for their weekly walk, seek comfort in food or alcohol, or reduce their commitment to an eating plan, telling themselves, *I'm too busy* or *I'll start next week*, and then they don't.

In order to avoid conflict, they may appear to agree to follow a certain weight-loss program but covertly undermine it. Visits to healthcare professionals may be "forgotten" or postponed. The energized step of a healthy Nine becomes a slow trudge.

Unhealthy

As weight loss stops, Nines can become increasingly resigned to being overweight and display a "what's the point?" attitude. They may ignore the pleas of loved ones or the warnings of health practitioners and become belligerent if pressured, interpreting the help offered as others trying to undermine their happiness. All the while, they may wishfully imagine the lighter body they are unable to find the discipline to achieve. They eat mindlessly and veg out in front of TV or the computer. Taking the path of least resistance, they may appear to go along with the idea to get fitter suggested to them, but avoid doing anything about it. This "going with the flow" approach can make self-development, which is usually a tough task, harder for Nines than other types.

Any changes to their routine suggested by a health professional or fitness instructor will be largely ignored (Like all instinctual types, they don't like being controlled). They become ever more slothful in body and mind, resigned to their weight and in complete denial regarding the reality of their state of health.

To become healthy on all levels, Nines need to understand that the way to true peace is not to avoid conflict but to connect with their own anger. Avoiding conflict often creates more conflict. They need to step up to the plate—not to eat its contents but to commit to the world: to be in it, rather than floating dreamily above it. They need to understand that asserting themselves is about engaging with life, and that this authenticity will attract others not offend them. To be present to themselves is to be present to life itself.

Summary

Nines are dreamers and optimists. It stands to reason, then, that they may have enthusiastic fantasies about losing weight fast, and when reality (and slow weight loss) hits and their expectations aren't met, they'll lose interest fast. They need encouragement and help along the way. As mentioned earlier, their hidden stress (from suppressed anger) needs to be expressed in some form of mindfulness-based exercise therapy. Yoga and tai chi are good for relaxing and focusing the mind. Also beneficial are craniosacral therapy, Body Stress Release (BSR), a form of neuro-muscular release bodywork that assists the muscles surrounding the spine in relaxing and releasing, and other biofeedback-type somatic therapies that get Nines in touch with their bodies. As a Nine's anger is released, the need to stuff it down with food should lessen.

Small steps will be helpful rather than unrealistic goals. It won't hurt to add a fun or community element as well, such as walking in a group or meeting for coffee after exercise. Even cutting out one unhealthy food source, such as sugar, or committing to one weekly exercise date, is a huge start.

"I agreed with myself to attend a certain yoga class once a week," one Nine told me. "I committed to it being non-negotiable. That way it became a habit. I just did it. Later, I added to the routine with other exercise commitments. Then I tackled my eating habits in the same way."

It's also important for Nines to learn that their opinions do count and to speak up for themselves—to stop checking out and instead, check in with how they feel about something and know how to express this. To sometimes say, "Harry, I know you'd prefer steak, but we've been to the steakhouse the last six times in a row. Maybe this time we could do what I want to do and eat sushi."

Small achievable commitments, easily implementable routines, exercising or being on a weight-loss program with others while also having fun are the way to go for a Nine. You do truly count. Nines will be inspired to change if there is the promise that doing so will create a more peaceful life, with others not harassing them. They want peace, so if they can see that by taking better care of themselves, others will niggle them less, they can make significant changes.

Conclusion

We've taken a literary stroll around the Enneagram types, through the eyes of our eating and exercise habits. Perhaps you found your type along the way, or maybe you're still pondering a few possibilities. That's fine. The journey to self is different for everyone and there are no prizes for getting to your type first.

Remember though, who you are is not limited to your type; rather, understanding your type is the first step to recognizing how we limit ourselves to the potential wholeness we all are. Through understanding our fixations and passions, we can liberate ourselves from them.

We all experience anger, fear, shame, feeling melancholy, guilt, envy, greed and a host of other emotions. They are not limited to any particular type, even if they may show up more often in some types than in others.

My grandfather used to say that the higher up the path of any religion you climb, the more the various paths converge towards the summit. The Enneagrams are not a religion, but the analogy holds true when we see that the more integrated we become, the greater access we have to all the aspects of all the types. All types then essentially meet as One.

It is also important to note that the journey to integration is full of hills and valleys. Just as we feel we are getting closer to the summit of our being, life throws a curved ball that has us careering down the slope into the less healthy aspects of ourselves. And that's okay, because we now have the tools to recognize what is happening. We can't take revenge, blame others or act out the host of disintegrated reactions without now being conscious of exactly what they are and what we are doing. The Enneagram has brought awareness to ourselves and much as it feels delicious at times to point fingers in self-righteous blame, we in our hearts know that that is not the higher road to take. Taking responsibility is the start of the road to personal power.

~

On a more personal note, I would love to reveal that I have shed further kilos since those lost in the early stages of writing this book, but I have not. That my 54 kg body has returned. It has not (or at least yet). What I have lost though, is the feeling of shame surrounding my body. You know the feeling of looking into the mirror and then wanting to look away fast? That feeling.

Being able to see my naked self now, with love, compassion, and immense gratefulness for the body that has brought me on my life's journey, is worth to me far more than the movement on any scale. There is an acceptance of who I am. What has altered physically though, through writing this book and the early days of research, is my general health – my blood sugar has normalised, as has my cholesterol and various other factors. So now, with purpose, gratitude, and deeper understanding, I believe I'm on the way – and so are you.

The Enneagram Quiz

This fun test is designed as a rough guide to your Enneagram type. Our Wings, the numbers we move toward or away from, whether we are Social, Sexual, or Self-Preservation types, and most importantly, our level of integration, will all affect how we reply to the questions, meaning that the test should give us an idea of the Enneagram area we need to look in, but not always the actual type.

The best way to find your type is to feel what type resonates most with you. Ask friends, family, colleagues, or partners for their opinions. Sometimes others see things of which we are unaware. Read other books on the Enneagram, explore the many on-line resources available and do some of the more in depth tests until you really feel you can relate to your type. Sometimes we are the type we are least drawn to.

For each of the following sentences circle the statement that resonates most with you, a, b, or c. Each of these statements corresponds to one of the nine Enneagram types. If none of the statements in a sentence apply to you skip that sentence.

1. At a buffet, I...
    a. would prefer something made especially for me
    b. employ a disciplined approach to food selection
    c. think, *Wow! So much choice!*

2. My philosophy regarding food is...
    a. eat or be eaten
    b. it's a reflection of my success to be seen eating the latest food trends
    c. cooking is love made visible

3. **My ideal restaurant is...**
    a. somewhere upmarket, new, and trendy
    b. romantic and unusual
    c. somewhere I've been before that's a safe bet for a good meal

4. **When it comes to leftovers, I...**
    a. cater carefully so that there seldom is wastage
    b. am thrilled—it'll save cooking again for days
    c. give them to the homeless

5. **When I am given an unusual dish, I...**
    a. am suspicious about its contents
    b. am excited to try something new
    c. can't wait to photograph and blog about it on Instagram

6. **When shopping, I look for...**
    a. things I can buy in bulk and thereby avoid unnecessary shopping trips
    b. whatever looks great, I just buy
    c. artisanal items that excite my love of good food

7. **When the food at a restaurant is disappointing, I...**
    a. complain – it's not acceptable
    b. say nothing – I don't make a fuss
    c. go into the kitchen to tell the chef

8. **Regarding conversation at the table with friends, I...**
    a. mostly keep quiet
    b. love telling a good story
    c. ask others about themselves

9. **I enjoy eating the same meal every lunchtime...**
    a. never – variety is the spice of life
    b. absolutely – then I don't have to think about it
    c. yes, it's less work

10.. **When it comes to dishing up food, I...**
   a. like to dish up for my partner
   b. choose what I want to eat
   c. enjoy my partner feeding me morsels

11. **When it comes to ordering at a restaurant, I...**
   a. choose what most people are having
   b. choose what will make me look good and sophisticated
   c. choose an expensive dish if I'm not paying

12. **I enjoy the type of food that's...**
   a. comforting
   b. that's ethically sourced - I enjoy doing what's right
   c. anything I don't have to prepare myself

13. **Presentation of a dish is...**
   a. not that important – I'm more concerned with the cleanliness of the cutlery
   b. unimportant to me, as long as there is lots of it and it tastes amazing
   c. very important to me – it's got to look beautiful

14. **I enjoy entertaining...**
   a. absolutely, it's a great way to make business contacts
   b. I don't
   c. I do, if I can decide what to make

15. **When it comes to dieting, I...**
   a. can never decide which diet is best
   b. set definite goals or targets for myself
   c. look for a friend who needs help sticking to their diet and team up with them

16. **If I have to choose a restaurant to go to with visiting colleagues, I...**
   a. plan a whole night's entertainment at various venues
   b. pick somewhere that's not too pricey – I don't want the office to think I'm wasting money.
   c. try to find somewhere that will make everyone happy

17. **When I shop, I...**
     a. always come home with some special sweet treats for family and colleagues
     b. usually have my partner do the daily grocery shop, but I enjoy hitting the malls occasionally and blowing a bunch of cash
     c. make a list, so as not to be tempted to buy what we don't really need

18. **I do yoga or would take it up because...**
     a. of its spiritual approach and focus on a deeper level of self-awareness
     b. of the slow pace of Yin, Hatha, or Restorative Yoga
     c. I enjoy perfecting the poses

19. **Competitive bodybuilding to me is...**
     a. incomprehensible
     b. about making my body my art
     c. a visible way to show off my goal of getting amazing pecs

20. **I prefer...**
     a. teamsports
     b. individual sports
     c. sports where I can excel

21. **I exercise because...**
     a. hey, I'll try anything, if it's fun
     b. I'm worried about my long-term health
     c. I want to support my friend/partner/colleague

22. **When it comes to winning, I...**
     a. don't know the meaning of "lose." If it ever happens, then revenge is on the cards.
     b. will do whatever it takes to win and achieve my goal
     c. am afraid that by winning, I will upset the other competitors

23. **In a team, I tend to focus more on...**
     a. the team's performance at the expense of my own
     b. my own achievement at the expense of the teams'
     c. the fact that I don't enjoy being part of a team

24. **I participate in teamsports because...**
    a. I enjoy leading my team to victory
    b. I love being one of the guys/gals
    c. it feels good to help my teammates improve

25. **I prefer to exercise on my own because...**
    a. I'm afraid that if I underperform I'll upset the rest of the team
    b. people drain me, and I enjoy time alone to ponder
    c. it's stressful if I perform badly to feel I've let the team down

26. **When I set myself an exercise goal, I...**
    a. normally achieve it – I'm a goal-oriented person
    b. mean to stick to it but get distracted and lazy
    c. find that there's often someone who needs my help, so I can't stick to it

27. **I don't exercise because...**
    a. I'm too caught up in my latest project
    b. I've never understood the desire to get hot and sweaty
    c. it starts off fun but then becomes routine and boring

28. **When I have an exercise plan, I...**
    a. stick to it rigidly
    b. vacillate between sticking to it and then not doing so
    c. stick to it if it's going to ensure I'm stronger and more likely to win

29. **My home is...**
    a. usually a mess – I never get round to tidying up
    b. warm and inviting
    c. a place with beautiful objects that I've selected carefully

30. **In my appearance, I aim to look...**
    a. cool and trendy
    b. flash – I enjoy having some bling
    c. different — maybe even a bit retro

Answer Key

Q1: a=4, b=1, c=7		Q16: a=7, b=1, c=9	
Q2: a=8, b=3, c=2		Q17: a=2, b=8, c=1	
Q3: a=3, b=4, c=6		Q18: a=4, b=9, c=1	
Q4: a=1, b=9, c=2		Q19: a=5, b=4, c=3	
Q5: a=6, b=7, c=4		Q20: a=6, b=5, c=3	
Q6: a=5, b=8, c=7		Q21: a=7, b=6, c=2	
Q7: a=1, b=9, c=8		Q22: a=8, b=3, c=9	
Q8: a=5, b=7, c=6		Q23: a=6, b=3, c=5	
Q9: a=7, b=5, c=9		Q24: a=8, b=6, c=2	
Q10: a=2, b=8, c=4		Q25: a=4, b=5, c=1	
Q11: a=9, b=3, c=5		Q26: a=3, b=9, c=2	
Q12: a=2, b=1, c=9		Q27: a=5, b=4, c=7	
Q13: a=1, b=8, c=4		Q28: a=1, b=6, c=8	
Q14: a=3, b=5, c=6		Q29: a=9, b=2, c=4	
Q15: a=6, b=3, c=2		Q30: a=7, b=8, c=4	

Use the answer key above to see which type applies to you for that sentence. (E.g. Q1: If you answered "a" then the answer key shows that "a" corresponds to a type Four, "b" to a type One and "c" to a type Seven.) Tally your totals for each type in the boxes below to see which type/s score the highest. This will give you an indication of what type you might be or which areas of the Enneagram you might want to look into.

Type 1: ☐   Type 4: ☐   Type 7: ☐

Type 2: ☐   Type 5: ☐   Type 8: ☐

Type 3: ☐   Type 6: ☐   Type 9: ☐

Acknowledgments

"No man or woman is an island."

Along the way I have had the honor to be taught by many teachers, some living and some long since passed on. Many have been authors themselves. Russ Hudson, in particular, whose workshops and writing, together with the late Don Riso, I found inspiring; Sandra Maitri; Pam Roux; Claudio Naranjo; Beatrice Chestnut; Helen Plamer; among others—thank you for sharing your insightful information and teachings with the world. I'm grateful, too, to the people I have interacted with, either as friends, pupils, or in the past, as clients. Each relationship has added both depth and richness to my experience of the Enneagram. Thank you, all.

To my editor, Nicky Leach, for saving me from myself and in so doing, making the book so much better and easier to read (and working through my comma fixation with a smile).

To Sabine Weeke and the team from Findhorn Press—your warmth and humor have been endearing, and it's been a pleasure working with you. Thanks also to my publishers for believing in me sufficiently to publish six of my books. That's a lot of positive reinforcement! Thank you from the bottom of my heart.

To my much-loved family, who have endured my absences with understanding and who have been insightful sounding boards for my ideas, as well as providing valuable input—thank you deeply, Anthony, Tess, and Taun, (supper will now be served…).

To Monika Afdeling (Mons), from the Nine Domains, who went through the book at its early stages and was wonderfully encouraging and supportive.

To the dietitians whose input I've sought over the past years—your patience is commendable, particularly Judith Johnson, who enjoyed the idea when I first shared it with her (and yes, I'm still on the green shakes).

To my friends and family: Ruth Bradburn, Glynis and Jamie Hart, Gareth and Coralie Bradburn, Lydia Carstens, Marianne de Jager, Clive Lucas, Terese le Merle Walther, Hazel Trehearn, Jenny Norman, Jenni Normand, Jeanine Nauta—thank you for being who you are.

And lastly, to the unseen support and inner guidance I have received along the path to completion of this book, which never fails to astound and humble me—my grateful acknowledgment.

Notes

Prologue

1. UCLA researchers report in the 2007 April issue of *American Psychologist*, the journal of the American Psychological Association. Traci Mann, UCLA associate professor of psychology and lead author of the study: "We found that the majority of people regained all the weight, plus more. Sustained weight loss was found only in a small minority of participants, while complete weight regain was found in the majority. Diets do not lead to sustained weight loss or health benefits for the majority of people."

   "Among those who were followed for fewer than two years, 23 percent gained back more weight than they had lost, while of those who were followed for at least two years, 83 percent gained back more weight than they had lost," Mann said. "One study found that 50 percent of dieters weighed more than 11 pounds over their starting weight five years after the diet," she said.

About the Enneagram

1. 2013–2014 NHANES survey of the National Centre for Health Statistics (NCHS).

2. 2011–12, around 60 percent of Australian adults were classified as overweight or obese, and more than 25 percent of these fell into the obese category (ABS 2012). In 2007, around 25 percent of children aged 2–16 were overweight or obese, with 6 percent classified as obese (DoHA 2008).

   A 2009 report by the Organisation for Economic Co-operation and Development (OECD) predicts that there will be continued increases in overweight and obesity levels across all age groups over the next decade in Australia, to around 66 percent of the population (Sassi et al. 2009).

3. Workshop in Cape Town with Russ Hudson, 2014.

4. The Law of Three is described by Gurdjieff as "the second fundamental cosmic law." This law states that every whole phenomenon is composed of three separate sources, which are *Active, Passive,* and *Reconciling* or *Neutral.* This law applies to everything in the *universe* and *humanity*, as well as all the *structures* and *processes.* The *Three Centers* in a human, which Gurdjieff said were the Intellectual Centre, the Emotional Centre, and the Moving Centre, are an expression of the Law of Three. Gurdjieff taught his students to think of the Law of Three forces as essential to transforming the *energy* of the *human being.* The process of transformation requires the three actions of *affirmation, denial,* and *reconciliation.* https://en.wikipedia.org/wiki/Fourth_Way#Basis_of_teachings

5. How the Law of Seven and Law of Three function together is said to be illustrated on the *Fourth Way Enneagram*, a nine-pointed symbol that is the central glyph

of Gurdjieff's system. According to Pyotr Demianovich Ouspensky, a Russian mathematician and major contributor to the early Enneagram work, "the Law of Three determines the character and nature of a vibration and the Law of Seven determines how vibrations develop, interact, and change. An octave is a repetitive motion. A succession of waves may be building up or dying away—forming an ascending or a descending octave. Each wave is similar but different to the one before and the one after. The Law of Seven also shows the points in the scale where the rate of increase or decrease of frequency of any vibration slows down. https://www.ouspenskytoday.org/wp/about-teaching-today/the-law-of-seven/

6. The terms "Social," "Sexual," and "Self-Preservation" were, I believe, originally coined by Claudio Naranjo. I first came across them, though, in the book *The Wisdom of the Enneagrams* by Don Richard Riso and Russ Hudson (Bantam Books, 1999).

7. Don Richard Riso and Russ Hudson. *The Wisdom of the Enneagrams.* (Bantam Books, 1999), p. 70.

8. The Riso / Hudson Levels of Development (LoD) referred to as "Healthy," "Average," and "Unhealthy" from the *Inner Critic* workshop given by Russ Hudson in Cape Town, 2013, as well as p. 106 and thereafter for each type in *The Wisdom of the Enneagrams* by Don Richard Riso and Russ Hudson.

Type One

1. Beatrice Chestnut. *The Complete Enneagram.* (She Writes Press, 2013), p. 403.

2. Don Richard Riso and Russ Hudson. *The Wisdom of the Enneagrams.* (Bantam Books, 1999), p. 351.

3. Riso, Hudson. *The Wisdom of the Enneagrams* (Bantam Books, 1999), p. 101.

4. Sandra Maitri. *The Spiritual Dimension of the Enneagram.* (Penguin Putnam Inc., 2001), p. 117.

5. *Keys to facilitating Enneagram Transformations for coaches, therapists, and change agents* – lecture by Ben Saltzman from the 2017 Enneagram Summit Global Lectures.

6. Riso, Hudson. *Understanding the Enneagram.* p. 157.

Type Two

1. The title used here is from The Enneagram Institute website (*www.enneagraminstitute*.com) and various books by Don Richard Riso and Russ Hudson.

2. Chestnut, *The Complete Enneagram.* p. 351.

3. Riso Richard, Hudson. *Personality Types* (Houghton Mifflin Company, 1996), p. 90-93.

4. Riso, Hudson. *The Wisdom of the Enneagrams.* p. 133.

5. Chestnut. *The Complete Enneagram.* p. 363.

6. Chestnut. *The Complete Enneagram.* p. 368.

7. Riso, Hudson. *The Wisdom of the Enneagrams.* p. 351.

8. There are regular episodes of "binge" eating, usually in private, of foods believed to be fattening and, therefore, in some way "forbidden" to someone wanting to control their weight. Foods typically eaten during a binge will include cookies, chocolate, potato chips, bowls of cereal, large amounts of toast with butter, french fries, cakes, tubs of ice cream, and so on. http://eating-disorders.org.uk/information/bulimia -nervosa-a-contemporary-analysis

9. *http://www.dietnosis.com/enneagram-types/enneagram-type-two/*. Although blame is widely accepted as a Type Two trait, Dr Scott M Harrington DO emphasizes how it affects performance: "Type Twos who are not currently exercising, may blame it on their family, work and social commitments."

Type Three

1. Riso, Hudson. *The Wisdom of the Enneagrams*, p. 153, and Helen Palmer. *The Enneagram in Love & Work,* p. 83.

2. http://www.dietnosis.com/enneagram-types/enneagram-type-three "They like to surround themselves with things that show their achievements or display photos of themselves with famous people."

3. https://www.health24.com/Lifestyle/Ageing-well/Surgical-procedures/butt-surgery -on-the-increase-in-america-20160229 Sourced Nov 2017

4. https://www.health24.com/Lifestyle/Ageing-well/Surgical-procedures/butt-surgery -on-the-increase-in-america-20160229 Sourced Nov 2017

5. https://trends.realself.com/2015/06/25/why-plastic-surgery-confidence-survey

6. Riso, Hudson. *The Wisdom of the Enneagrams*. p. 351.

7. From *World Psychiatry* https://www.ncbi.nlm.nih.gov/pmc/articles/PMC4911756 accessed June 2017.

8. Riso, Hudson. *The Wisdom of the Enneagrams*. p. 156.

9. http://www.independent.co.uk/life-style/health-and-families/health-news/bigorexia -what-is-muscle-dysmorphia-and-how-many-people-does-it-affect-10511964.html. Tod, D., Edwards, C., & Cranswick, I. (2016). Muscle dysmorphia: Current insights. *Psychology Research and Behavior Management, 9*, 10. Accessed 16/11/2017 I discovered the word "bigorexia" on this fascinating website: http://www.dietnosis .com/enneagram-types/enneagram-type-three. Accessed: August 2017.

10. *Keys to Facilitating Enneagram Transformations for Coaches, Therapists, and Change Agents* – lecture by Ben Saltzman from the 2017 Enneagram Global Summit Lectures. Saltzman was using the reference here in relation to therapists, life skill coaches, and change agents, in general, but it equally applies in my understanding to dietitians, doctors, and sports coaches.

11. I first came across the idea that Threes, as they became less healthy, lose touch with what it is they really want to be or do with their lives at the Inner Critic workshop given by Russ Hudson in Cape Town in 2013.

Type Four

1. https://en.wikipedia.org/wiki/Hipster_(contemporary_subculture)

2. Riso, Hudson. *Personality Types*. p. 167-169.

3. Riso, Hudson. *The Wisdom of the Enneagrams*. p. 351.

4. Beatrice Chestnut. *The Complete Enneagram*. p. 272.

5. Ben Saltzman. *Keys to Facilitating Enneagram Transformations for Coaches, Therapists, and Change Agents* – lecture by from the 2017 Enneagram Global Summit Lectures.

Type Five

1. This is from a 2014 workshop *The Nine Journeys*, with Russ Hudson in Cape Town.

2. Mary Horsley. *The Enneagram of Spirit*. p. 42. (Barron's Educational Series inc., 2005.)

3. https://www.starchefs.com/features/ten-international-pioneers/recipe-sound-of-the -sea-heston-blumenthal.shtml. Sound of the Sea recipe. Chef Heston Blumenthal of The Fat Duck – Bray, England. Adapted by StarChefs.com. Accessed Feb. 2017.

4. Claudio Naranjo. *Character and Neurosis*. (Gateways/IDHHB, INC., 1994) p. 66 "This is a fearful grasping, implying a fantasy that letting go would result in catastrophic depletion. Behind the hoarding impulse there is, we may say, an experience of impending impoverishment."

5. Riso, Hudson. *The Wisdom of the Enneagrams*. p. 351.

6. Chestnut. *The Complete Enneagram*. p. 232.

7. Claudio Naranjo. *Character and Neurosis*. p. 86.

8. Riso,Hudson. *At-a-Glance Personality Elements*. Chart.

Type Six

1. This is from a 2014 workshop *The Nine Journeys*, with Russ Hudson in Cape Town.

2. Riso, Hudson. *Personality Types*. p. 236.

3. Riso, Hudson. *The Wisdom of the Enneagrams*. p. 253.

4. Dr. Scott Harrington on Food Decision Factors, http://www.dietnosis.com /enneagram-types/enneagram-type-six, accessed in February 2017.

5. From a 2013 workshop, *The Inner Critic*, with Russ Hudson in Cape Town.

6. Dr. Scott Harrington on Enneagram Type 6 at Home, http://www.dietnosis.com /enneagram-types/enneagram-type-six.

7. Chestnut. *The Complete Enneagram*. p. 31-32.

8. Chestnut. The Complete Enneagram. p. 32.

9. Chestnut. The Complete Enneagram. p. 207.

10. Riso, Hudson. *The Wisdom of the Enneagrams*. p. 351.

11. Sandra Maitri. *The Spiritual Dimension of the Enneagram*. (Penguin Putnam Inc. 2001.) p. 70.

12. This concept of straying gurus came to mind after reading the book *Do You Need a Guru?* by Mariana Caplan (Thorsons, 2002), in which she describes her exploits with various "gurus," many of whom expected sexual favors in return for "enlightenment."

13. Dr. Scott Harrington, Favorite Exercises on http://www.dietnosis.com/enneagram-types/enneagram-type-six/. accessed in September 2017.

14. From the movie *'Kissed by God'* on the life of Andy Irons by Tetron Gravity Research.

Type Seven

1. Riso, Hudson. *Discovering Your Personality Type*. p. 146.

2. Riso, Hudson, *The Wisdom of the Enneagrams*. p. 279.

3. *Ready, Steady, Cook* was a BBC cooking program that first aired in 1994.

4. Riso, Hudson. *The Wisdom of the Enneagrams*. p. 351.

5. Riso, Hudson. *Personality Types*. p. 265.

6. Naranjo describes it as a "passion for pleasure." *Character and Neurosis*. p. 151.

7. Ben Saltzman. *Keys to Facilitating Enneagram Transformations for Coaches, Therapists and Change Agents* – lecture by from the 2017 Enneagram Global Summit Lectures.

Type Eight

1. Song played as an example of an Eight at *The Enneagram One Day Workshop* presented in 2011 by Barry Coltham.

2. Riso, Hudson. *The Wisdom of the Enneagrams*. p. 227.

3. Riso, Hudson. *The Wisdom of the Enneagrams*. p. 293.

4. As an artist myself, and being married to an artist, I have found many of my patrons to be Type Eights with Nine Wings.

5. Katherine Chernick Fauvre. Enneastyle: The Nine Languages and Personal Presentations of the Nine Enneagram Types, from the Enneagram Global Summit Lectures June 2017. p. 7.

6. Dr. Scott Harrington, Enneagram Type Eight Fashion http://www.dietnosis.com/enneagram-types/enneagram-type-eight/. accessed Nov. 2016.

7. Claudio Naranjo. Character and Neurosis. p. 146.

8. Riso, Hudson. *The Wisdom of the Enneagrams*. p. 351.

9. Jerome Wagner, *Integrating Our Inner Polarities* From a 2013 workshop, with Russ Hudson, *The Inner Critic*, in Cape Town.

10. Ben Saltzman, *Keys to Facilitating Enneagram Transformations for Coaches, Therapists, and Change Agents* – lecture by from the 2017 Enneagram Global Summit Lectures. p. 9.

11. Jerome Wagner. *Integrating Our Inner Polarities* – lecture by from the 2017 Enneagram Global Summit Lectures. p. 11.

12. Ben Saltzman, *Keys to Facilitating Enneagram Transformations for Coaches, Therapists, and Change Agents* – lecture by from the 2017 Enneagram Global Summit Lectures.

Type Nine

1. Riso, Hudson. *The Wisdom of the Enneagrams.* p. 23.

2. Riso, Hudson. *The Wisdom of the Enneagrams.* p. 351.

3. http://www.bariatric-solutions.com/wDeutsch/for-patients/adiposity/physiology -and-pathophysiology.php, sourced Nov 2017

NOTE: There are some references to Riso/Hudson Type names: Achiever (p. 55), Helper (p. 43), and Peacemaker (p. 154). These names are copyright of The Enneagram Institute.*

Bibliography

Aldridge, Susan. *Seeing Red and Feeling Blue*. London: Arrow Books, 2001.

Atkinson, Mark. *The Mind Body Bible*. London: Piatkus, 2008.

Bays, Brandon. *The Journey*. London: Thorsons, 1999.

Borysenko, Joan. *A Woman's Spiritual Journey*. London: Piatkus, 2000.

Campling, Matthew. *The 12-Type Enneagram*. London: Watkins, 2015.

Caplan, Mariana. *Do You Need a Guru?* London: Thorsons, 2002.

Chestnut, Beatrice, PhD. *The Complete Enneagram*. Berkeley, CA: She Writes Press, 2013.

Chopra, Deepak. *How to Know God*. London: Rider Books, 2001.

———. *Overcoming Addictions*. London: Random House, 2001.

Cwynar, Eva. *The Fatigue Solution*. Cape Town, South Africa: Hay House, 2012.

D'Adamo, Peter, with Catherine Whitney. *The Eat Right Diet*. London: Century Books, 1998.

Davis, William. Wheat Belly. New York: Rodale Books, 2014.

Dethlefsen, Thorwald and Rüdiger Dahlke. *The Healing Power of Illness*. Shaftesbury, UK: Element Books, 1990.

Diamond, Marilyn and Harvey. *Fit for Life*. London. Bantam, 1998.

Dukan, Pierre. *The Dukan Diet*. London: Hodder & Stoughton, 2010.

Evans, Philip. *The Family Medical Reference Book*. London: Time Warner, 2003.

Ford, Debbie. *The Dark Side of the Light Chasers*. London: Hodder & Stoughton, 2001.

Fortune, Dion. *The Mystical Qabalah*. Wellingborough: The Aquarian Press, 1987.

Goldin, Paul. *Lose Weight Think Slim*. London: Boxtree, 1995.

Govindji, Azmina and Nina Puddefoot. *GI Point Diet*. London: Vermilion, 2004.

Hanh, Thich Nhat. *The Heart of the Buddha's Teachings*. Berkeley, CA: Broadway Books, 1998.

Hay, Louise. *Heal Your Body*. Cape Town, South Africa: Hay House/ Paradigm Press, 1993.

Horsley, Mary. *The Enneagram for the Spirit*. New York: Barron's Educational Series inc., 2005.

Joffe, Yael and Judith Johnson and Alex Royal. *Genes to Plate*. Cape Town, South Africa: Impact Clinics, 2017.

Johnson, Robert A. *Owning Your Own Shadow*. San Francisco, CA: HarperCollins, 1993.

Judith, Anodea. *Eastern Body, Western Mind*. Berkeley, CA: Celestial Arts, 1996.

Kamphuis, Albert. *Egowise Leadership & the Nine Creating Forces of the Innovation Circle*. Self-published. Netherlands: Egowise Leadership Academy, 2011.

Kornfield, Jack. *A Path with a Heart*. New York: Bantam, 1993.

Lipton, Bruce H. *The Biology of Belief*. Santa Rosa, CA: Mountain of Love/ Elite Books, 2005.

Lytton, Edward Bulwer. *Zanoni: A Rosicrucian Tale*. Whitefish, MT: Kessinger Publishing.

Maitri, Sandra. *The Spiritual Dimension of the Enneagram*. New York: Penguin Putnam Inc., 2001.

———. *The Enneagram of Passions and Virtues*. New York: Penguin Random House. 2009.

McKeith, Gillian. *You Are What You Eat*. New York: Plume/Penguin, 2006.

McKenna, Paul. *I Can Make You Thin*. London: Transworld, 2005.

Millman, Dan. *The Life You Were Born to Live*. Novato, CA: HJ Kramer in a joint venture with New World Library, 1993.

Mindell, Earl. *The Vitamin Bible*. London: Arlington Books, 1992.

Murphy, Joseph. *The Power of Your Subconscious Mind*. New York: The Penguin Group, 2008.

Myss, Caroline. *Anatomy of the Spirit*. London: Bantam, 1998.

———. *Why People Don't Heal And How They Can*. London. Bantam, 1998.

Naranjo, Claudio. *Character and Neurosis*. Nevada City, CA: Gateways/ IDHHB, Inc. 2003.

Noakes, Tim, Sally-Ann Creed, and Jonno Proudfoot. *The Real Meal Revolution*. London: Robinson Publications Ltd., 2015.

Palmer, Helen. *The Enneagram in Love & Work.* New York: Harper One, 1995.

_____ . *The Enneagram: Understanding Yourself and Others in Your Life.* New York: Harper One, 1991.

Pearson, Carol S. *Awakening the Heroes Within.* New York: HarperCollins, 1991.

_____ . *The Heroes Within.* New York: HarperCollins, 1998.

Peirce Thompson, Susan. *Bright Line Eating.* New York: Hay House, 2017.

Riso, Don Richard and Russ Hudson. *The Wisdom of the Enneagram.* New York: Bantam Books, 1999.

_____ . *Understanding the Enneagram.* Rev. ed. Boston, MA: Houghton Mifflin Company, 2000.

_____ . *Discovering Your Personality Type.* Boston, MA: Houghton Mifflin Company, 2003.

_____ . *Personality Types.* Boston, MA: Houghton Mifflin Company, 1996.

Roth, Geneen. *Woman Food and God.* London: Simon & Schuster, 2010.

Shapiro, Debbie. *Your Body Speaks Your Mind.* London: Piatkus, 1996.

Shealy Norman C. and Caroline Myss. *The Creation of Health.* Walpole, NH: Stillpoint Publishing, 1998.

Stone, Joshua David. *Soul Psychology.* New York: Ballantine Wellspring, 1999.

Surya Das, Lama. *Awakening to the Sacred.* New York: Broadway Books, 1999.

Thondup, Tukulu. *The Healing Power of the Mind.* Boston, MA: Shambhala Publications, 1996.

Tolle, Eckhart. *The Power of Now.* London: Hodder & Stoughton, 2005.

Trattler, Ross. *Better Health Through Natural Healing.* New York: McGraw-Hill, 1997.

Zuercher, Suzanne. *Enneagram Spirituality.* Notre Dame, IN: Ave Maria Press, 1992.

About the Author

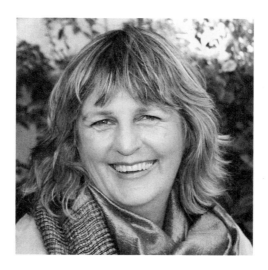

Ann Gadd is an accredited Enneagram practitioner (iEQ9 certified), holistic therapist, artist, workshop facilitator, author, and journalist. An avid, long-term student of the Enneagram, she offers Enneagram workshops for beginners and advanced students. The author of 21 books, including *The Girl Who Bites Her Nails*, *The A – Z of Common Habits*, and *Finding Your Feet*, Ann lives in Cape Town, South Africa.

FINDHORN PRESS

Life-Changing Books

Learn more about us and our books at
www.findhornpress.com

For information on the Findhorn Foundation:
www.findhorn.org